ANALYZER OF MEDICAL · BIOLOGICAL WORDS

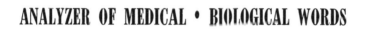

ANALYZER
of
MEDICAL · BIOLOGICAL WORDS

A Clarifying Dissection of Medical Terminology, Showing How It Works, for
Medics, Paramedics, Students, and Visitors
from Foreign Countries

By

J. E. SCHMIDT, M.D.

Author of Paramedical Dictionary; Visual Aids
for Paramedical Vocabulary; Structural Units of
Medical and Biological Terms; English Word
Power for Physicians; English Speech for
Foreign Students; English Idioms and Ameri-
canisms for Foreign Professionals

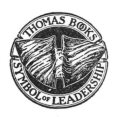

CHARLES C THOMAS · PUBLISHER
Springfield · Illinois · U.S.A.

Published and Distributed Throughout the World by

CHARLES C THOMAS • PUBLISHER

BANNERSTONE HOUSE

301-327 East Lawrence Avenue, Springfield, Illinois, U.S.A.

© *1973, by* J. E. SCHMIDT

ISBN 0-398-02682-3

Library of Congress Catalog Card Number: 74-88454

With THOMAS BOOKS *careful attention is given to all details of manufacturing and design. It is the Publisher's desire to present books that are satisfactory as to their physical qualities and artistic possibilities and appropriate for their particular use.* THOMAS BOOKS *will be true to those laws of quality that assure a good name and good will.*

Printed in the United States of America

C-2

INTRODUCTION

THE purpose of the book is to acquaint the reader with the "anatomy" and "histology," as it were, of the medical and biological vocabulary. The understanding of the structure of a word makes it much easier to appreciate and to remember its meaning. It is as useful to understand the combining forms forming a word as it is to recognize the letters of which it is composed—perhaps even more so.

With few exceptions, the vocabularies of the biological sciences are derived from the Latin and the Greek languages. Some terms are taken literatim from the original Greek or Latin; others are modified, more or less. But most biological terms are compound structures, the sum of two, three, or more Greek or Latin words that have been modified or etymologically shaped to facilitate their fusion and to shorten as much as possible the resulting chain structure. The modified components of a compound word are known as *stems* and *roots*, depending on how much remains of the original word. The stems and roots are the principal structural units of the biological terminology. They may be envisioned as bricks, or stones, or cinder blocks of an architectural structure.

Aside from these meaningful roots or stems—often referred to as "combining forms"—compound words often contain smaller particles, seldom or never used alone, which add meaning or semantic direction to the more imposing superstructure or main body of the term. Such a small particle is known as a *prefix* when it is attached to the beginning of a word, as the *a* in *avitaminosis*, an abnormal condition resulting from a lack of vitamins. A particle which is situated at the end of a word is known as a *suffix,* as the -*ist* in *physicist.* In this case it indicates "a person who. . . ."

A still smaller structural unit, having no meaning at all, is used as a linguistic mortar to join meaningful units, mainly for the sake of euphony or ease of articulation. When combining forms of Latin origin are joined, the particle or "cement" is generally an *i.* In the case of Greek combining forms, the joiner is usually an *o.* An example of the former is *bronch-i-loquy.* An example of the latter is *phren-o-logy.*

HOW TO DISARTICULATE WORDS

The knowledge that a given biological term is a fusion product composed of two or more classical stems helps in the analysis, but it is not enough. To disarticulate a word one must be able to discern its sutures or seams, so that the cleavage will result in meaningful particles. To imbue the reader with this essential knowledge, the following text presents a dissection of the more representative biological terms, showing their disjointed forms and the stems, roots, prefixes, suffixes, and joining particles which partake in the structural scheme. The reader who will assimilate the expertise thus presented will have no difficulty in analyzing the thousands of medical and other biological terms not treated specifically in this book.

THE PLAN OF PRESENTATION

The material in this book is arranged alphabetically on the basis of the stems or roots. These combining forms are followed by a brief statement with regard to their origin and their meaning in the source words. It should be noted that the meaning of a combining form as a component of a biological term is often somewhat different from the meaning of the source word. Each combining form or group of combining forms is followed by an example of usage. The biological term used as an example is given in a disarticulated form, so that the reader can see at once the two or more component parts. The example is briefly defined, and the definition is followed by an explanation as to meaning and source of all the combining forms used in the sample words. In those cases in which a combining form is taken from an inflected form of the source word, usually the genitive case, the inflected word is also given.

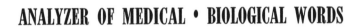

ANALYZER OF MEDICAL · BIOLOGICAL WORDS

A

a- ... an- ... Greek prefixes meaning *without, not, negative, separation from, absence of*. Note: *a* is used before consonants; *an* is used before vowels.

a-geus-ia. Lack of the sense of taste. / a (without) / geusis (G. taste) / ia (a noun-forming suffix used in names of *disorders*).

an-orex-ia. Absence of appetite for food. / an (without) / orexis (G. appetite) / ia (a noun-forming suffix used in names of *disorders*).

ab- ... A Latin prefix, based on *ab* (from), meaning *from, off, away from*.

ab-duct. To draw or move away from the midline. / ab / ducere (L. to lead).

abdomin- ... abdomino- ... Combining forms referring to the *abdomen*, derived from the Latin *abdomen* (genit. *abdominis*), the *belly*. Note that the spelling of the combining forms is based on the genitive, i.e. it is abdomin-, not abdomen-.

abdomin-alg-ia. Pain in the abdomen. / abdomin / algos (G. pain) / ia (a suffix used to form nouns).

abdomin-o-scop-y. Examination of the abdomen, especially the interior. / abdomin / o (a word-joining particle) / skopein (G. to view) / y (a suffix forming nouns).

3

-able . . . An adjective-forming suffix, from the Latin *-abilis,* meaning *able to, suitable for, characterized by, capable of being, tending to.*

palp-able. Capable of being perceived by touch. / palpare (L. to touch) / able.

ac- . . . A prefix having the same meaning and uses as the Latin *ad* (meaning *to, toward, near, together*), but used before the letters *c* and *q.*

ac-commodate. Of the eye, to become adjusted for a particular distance. / ad (to) / commodare (L. to fit).

-ac . . . An adjective-forming suffix, from the Latin *-acus,* meaning *characteristic of, pertaining to, affected by, having.*

celi-ac. Pertaining to the abdominal cavity. / koilia (G. abdomen) / ac.

-ac . . . A noun-forming suffix, from the Latin *acus,* meaning *a person affected by a specific condition.*

hemo-phili-ac. A person affected by hemophilia. / haima (G. blood) / philein (G. to love) / ac.

-aceous . . . A suffix, derived from the Latin *aceus* (of the nature of), used to form adjectives meaning *like, of the nature of, producing, belonging to, characterized by.*

membran-aceous. Like, or of the nature of, a membrane. / membrana (L. of membrane) / aceus (of the nature of).

acet- . . . **aceto-** . . . Combining forms, derived from the Latin *acetum* (vinegar), referring to *vinegar, acetic acid,* and other *acids.*

acet-ic. Like vinegar; pertaining to vinegar; involving acetic acid. / acet / ic (an adjective forming suffix designating a characteristic).

Aceto-bacter. A genus of microorganisms capable of producing vinegar or a vinegarlike fluid. / acet / o (a joining particle) /

baktron (G. a staff). *Note:* the "staff" refers to the shape of the microorganism.

-acid ... acidi- ... acido- ... Combining forms, derived from the Latin *acidus* (sour), used to designate *acid, sourness.*

hyper-acid-ity. A condition of excessive acidity, especially in the stomach. / hyper (G. above) / acid / ity (a suffix denoting a specified condition).

acido-phil-ic. Readily stained by acid dyes: fond of acid. / acido /philein (G. to love) / ic (a suffix forming adjectives designating certain characteristics).

-acou- ... -acous- ... acoustico- ... acousto- ... Greek combining forms, from *akouein* (to hear), *akoustikos* (pertaining to hearing), referring to *hearing.*

an-acous-ia. Absence of hearing; inability to hear. / an (without) / akoustikos / ia (a noun-forming suffix used in names of *diseases*).

acro- ... A Greek combining form, from *akros* (at the point or end), meaning *end, tip, extremity, limb.*

aoro ger-ia. A premature aging of the skin of the extremities. / akros / geras (G. old age) / ia (a noun-forming suffix used in names of *disorders*).

actin- ... actini- ... actino- ... Greek combining forms, from *aktis*, genit. *aktinos* (ray), meaning *ray, beam.*

actini-form. Resembling a ray or rays. / aktinos / forma (L. shape, form).

acu- ... A Latin combining form, from *acus* (needle), meaning *needle, pointed object.*

acu-puncture. The practice of piercing parts of the body with needles for the relief of pain or in the treatment of disease. / acus / punctura (L. a piercing).

-acy . . .   A noun-forming suffix, from the Latin *-acia*, denoting *condition, quality, status*.

lun-acy. Insanity; mental derangement. / luna (L. moon) / acy.

ad- . . .   A Latin prefix meaning *to, together, toward, near*. *Note: ad* becomes *ac* before the letters *c* and *q, af* before *f, ag* before *g, al* before *l, an* before *n, ap* before *p, ar* before *r, as* before *s, at* before *t*.

ad-stern-al. Toward the sternum. / ad (toward) / sternon (G. breastbone) / al (an adjective-forming suffix denoting a *quality*).

-ad . . .   A suffix, from the Latin *ad* (to), meaning *to, toward, in the direction of*.

cephal-ad. Toward the head. / kephale (G. head) / ad (toward).

-aden- . . .   **adeni-** . . .   **adeno-** . . .   Greek combining forms, from *aden*, genit. *adenos* (gland), meaning *gland*.

peri-aden-itis. Inflammation of the tissues surrounding a gland. / peri (G. around) / aden / itis (a suffix indicating *inflammation*).

adip- . . .   **adipo-** . . .   Latin combining forms, from adeps (fat), genit. adipis, referring to *fat, suet*.

adip-ec-tom-y. Excision of layers or masses of fat. / adipis / ek (G. out) / temnein (G. cut) / y (a noun-forming suffix indicating an *action*).

-aer- . . .   **aeri-** . . .   **-aero-** . . .   Combining forms, derived from the Greek *aer* (genit. *aeros*), air, having a reference to *air, gas, atmosphere*.

aer-ate. To supply with air; to charge with gas. / aer (air, gas) / ate (a verb-forming suffix).

aeri-fer-ous. Carrying or conveying air. / aeri (air) / ferre (L. bear) / ous (an adjective-forming suffix).

af- ... A prefix having the same uses as the Latin *ad* (meaning *to, toward, near, together*), but used before the letter *f*.

af-ferent. Conveying toward a specified structure. / ad (toward) / ferre (L. to bear).

ag- ... A prefix having the same uses as the Latin *ad* (meaning *to, toward, near, together*), but used (instead of *ad*) before the letter *g*.

ag-glutin-ate. To clump. / ad (together) / glutinare (L. to glue) / ate (a verb-forming suffix meaning *to become*).

-age ... A noun-forming suffix, from the Latin *-aticum*, denoting an *act, state, condition, service*.

drain-age. The act of drawing off, as exudate. / dreinen (Middle English, to strain off) / age.

-agogue ... A Greek suffix, from *agogos* (leading), meaning *inducing, inciting, stimulating, leading*.

galact-agogue. A substance which stimulates the production of milk in the breast. / gala, genit. galaktos (G. milk) / agogos.

agro- ... A Greek combining form, from *agros* (field), referring to *agriculture, fields*.

agro-bio-logy. The study of plants in relation to the factors which determine yields. / agros / bios (G. life) / logia (G. science, from *logos*, word, study).

al- ... A prefix having the same uses as the Latin *ad* (meaning *to, toward, near, together*), but used instead of *ad* before the letter *l*.

al-ligat-ion. A method for mixing medicinal fluids. / ad (together) / ligare, ligatus (L. to bind) / ion (a noun-forming suffix denoting a *process*).

-al ... A noun-forming suffix, from the Latin *-alis*, meaning a thing or a being having a particular characteristic, an act of doing something.

per-enni-al. A plant growing for three or more years. / per (L. through) / annus (L. year) / al.

-al ...   An adjective-forming suffix, from the Latin *-alis,* meaning *pertaining to, characterized by.*

hyster-ic-al. Characterized by hysteria. / hystera (G. the womb, once regarded as the cause of hysteria) / ic (pertaining to) / al.

alb- ...   albi- ...   albo- ...   albu- ...   Latin combining forms, from *albus* (white), meaning *white.*

alb-ation. An abnormal whitening of a tissue or structure. albus / ation (a noun-forming suffix denoting a *process*).

albumin- ...   albumini- ...   albumino- ...   Latin combining forms, from *albumen* (white of an egg), referring to the protein *albumin.*

albumini-par-ous. Producing albumin. / albumen / parere (L. bring forth) / ous (a Latin adjective-forming suffix meaning *marked by*).

alge- ...   algesi- ...   -algia ...   algo- ...   Greek combining forms, from *algos* (pain), meaning *pain, ache.*

alge-don-ic. Pertaining to a sensation of pleasure and pain. / algos / hedone (G. pleasure) / ic (an adjective-forming suffix meaning *pertaining to*).

all- ...   allo- ...   Greek combining forms, from *allos* (other), meaning *other, another, reversal, abnormal.*

all-erg-y. Abnormal reaction or work. / allos / ergon (G. work) / y (a noun-forming suffix denoting an *action*).

alti- ...   alto- ...   Latin combining forms, from *altus* (high), meaning *high, height.*

alti-metr-y. The measurement of height or altitude. / altus / metron (G. measure) / y (a noun-forming suffix denoting an *action*).

alveol-...   alveolo-... Combining forms, derived from the Latin *alveolus* (small hollow), referring to a *socket, small cavity, alveolus.*

alveol-itis. Inflammation of a tooth socket. / alveol (socket) / itis (inflammation).

alveolo-plasty. Plastic operation on a tooth socket or on the bone supporting the teeth. / alveolo / plassein (G. to form or shape).

amphi-...   ampho-... Combining forms, derived from the Greek *amphi* (on both sides), meaning *both, both sides, double.*

amphi-bious. Living both on land and in water. / amphi (both, of two kinds) / bios (G. life).

ampho-philic. Staining readily with both acid and basic dyes / ampho / philein (G. to love).

amyl-...   amylo-... Greek combining forms, from *amylon* (starch), referring to *starch.*

amyl-ase. An enzyme which aids in the splitting of starch. / amylon / ase (a suffix denoting an enzyme).

an-... prefix having the same uses as the Latin *ad* (meaning *to, together, near, toward*), but used instead of *ad* before the letter *n.*

an-nex. To add on or attach. / ad (to) / nectere, nexus (L. bind).

ana-... Greek prefix, from *ana* (up), meaning *up, upward, again, excessive.*

ana-bol-ism. The process of building up of complex substances in the body. / ana (up) / bole (G. a throw) / ism (a noun-forming suffix indicating a *process*).

-andr-...   andri-...   andro-... Greek combining forms, from *aner*, genit. *andros* (man), meaning *man, male, masculinity.*

andro-gyn-ism. A form of female pseudohermaphroditism. / andros / gyne (G. woman) / ism (a noun-forming suffix indicating a condition).

anemo-... A Greek combining form, from *anemos* (wind), meaning *wind, draft.*

anemo-phobia. An abnormal fear of winds or drafts. / anemos / phobos (G. fear).

angi-... **angio-...** Greek combining forms, from *angeion* (vessel), referring to a *blood vessel, lymph vessel.*

angio-spasm. A spasm of a blood vessel. / angeion / spasmos (G. spasm).

ankyl-... **ankylo-...** Combining forms, derived from the Greek *ankylos* (crooked), meaning *bent, curved, looped, crooked.*

ankyl-osis. An abnormal adhesion of the bones of a joint. / ankyl (crooked) / osis (an abnormal condition).

ankylo-blepharon. An abnormal adhesion of the edges of the eyelids. / ankylo / blepharon (G. eyelid).

ankyl-... **ankylo-...** Greek combining forms, from *ankylosis* (stiffening), meaning *immobility, adhesion, consolidation, ankylosis.*

ankylo-dactyl-ia. Adhesion of the fingers or toes. / ankylosis / daktylos (G. finger, toe) / ia (a Latin noun-forming suffix used in names of *disorders*).

-ant... 1. An adjective-forming suffix, from the Latin *-antem*, meaning *having the characteristics of.* 2. A noun-forming suffix meaning *one who, that which.*

re-sist-ant. Offering resistance or opposition. / re (L. back) / sistere (L. to set) / ant.

fumig-ant. A substance whose vapors kill insects, rodents, etc. / fumigare (L. to smoke) / ant.

ant- ... anti- ...   Prefixes, derived from the Greek *anti* (against), implying *opposite, reverse, opposed to, instead, against.*

ant-agonist. A muscle which acts counter to another muscle; one who opposes. / ant (against) / agonizesthai (G. to struggle).

anti-biotic. A substance destroying or arresting the growth of microorganisms. / anti (against) / biotikos (G. of life).

ante- ...   A prefix, derived from the Latin *ante* (before), meaning *prior, in front, forward, before.*

ante-febrile. Occurring before the onset of fever. / ante (prior) / febris (L. fever). *Note:* the suffix *ile* designates a condition.

ante-cede. To come before / ante / cedere (L. come, go).

anthrop- .,,   anthropo ...   Greek combining forms, from *anthropos* (man), referring to *man, human being.*

anthrop-oid. Resembling man. / anthropos / eides (G. having form of).

antr- ...   antro- ...   Combining forms, derived from the Greek *antron* or the Latin *antrum* (a cave), referring to a *sinus, antrum, cavity.*

antr-odynia. Pain in a sinus or antrum. / antr (sinus) / odyne (G. pain). *Note:* the suffix *ia* is used to form nouns.

antro-stomy. The surgical formation of an opening in an antrum or sinus. / antro / stoma (G. mouth, opening).

ap- ...   A prefix having the same uses as the Latin *ad (to, toward, near, together),* but used instead of *ad* before the letter *p.*

ap-pend-age. A subordinate structure. / ad (to) / pendere (L. to suspend) / age (a noun-forming suffix denoting a *structure* and its *role*).

-aph- ...   haphe- ...   Greek combining forms, from *haphe* (touch), referring to *touch, perception of touch.*

hypo-aph-ia. Decreased sensitivity to touch. / hypo (less than normal) / haphe / ia (a noun-forming suffix used in names of *disorders*).

apo- ... A Greek prefix, based on *apo* (from), meaning *from, separation from, derivation from.*

apo-morphine. An alkaloid derived from morphine. / apo / morphine.

aqua- ... **aquat-** ... **aque-** ... Latin combining forms, from *aqua* (water) and *aquaticus* (watery), referring to *water, fluid.*

aque-duct. A conduit conveying water; an anatomical canal. / aquae (genit. of *aqua*) / ducere (L. to lead), past participle *ductus.*

ar- ... A prefix having the same uses as the Latin *ad* (*to, toward, near, together*), but used instead of *ad* before the letter *r.*

ar-rect-or. A muscle which raises something. / ad (toward) / regere (L. make upright), past participle *rectus* (straight) / or (a suffix denoting a thing that does).

-ar ... An adjective-forming suffix, from the Latin *-aris,* meaning *like, of the nature of.*

fibrill-ar. Resembling, or composed of, fibrils. / fibrilla (L. a small fiber) / ar.

-arachn- ... **arachno-** ... Greek combining forms, from *arachne* (spider), referring to *slenderness, spider, spider's web.*

sub-arachn-oid. Beneath the arachnoid membrane. / sub (beneath) / arachne (spider's web, in allusion to the delicate structure of the membrane) / eides (G. having the form of).

arbor- ... **arbori-** ... Latin combining forms, from *arbor* (a tree), referring to *a tree, treelike structure.*

arbor-ization. The formation of a treelike structure, as of blood vessels. / arbor / ization (a noun-forming suffix denoting *an act, process*).

arch-... **arche-**... **archi-**... Greek combining forms, from *archos* (ruler, first man), meaning *original, first, primitive, beginning.*

arche-type. An original type; prototype. / archos / typos (G. model).

archo-... A Greek combining form, from *archos* (rectum, anus), referring to the *rectum, anus.*

archo-cele. A hernia of the rectum. / archos / kele (G. hernia).

-archy... A Greek terminal combining form, from *archein* (to rule), meaning *a ruling, that which is ruled.*

matri-archy. A social organization dominated by the mother. / mater (L. mother), genit. *matris* / archia, archein.

-arium... A noun-forming suffix, from the Latin *-arius*, referring to a *place used for a particular purpose.*

sanit-arium. An institution for the care of convalescents and the chronically ill. / sanitas (L. health) / arium.

arter-... **arteri-**... **arterio-**... Combining forms, derived from the Latin *arteria* (windpipe, artery), referring to *arteries* or an *artery. Note:* the ancient namemakers believed that the arteries conveyed air.

arter-itis. Inflammation of an artery. / arter (artery) / itis (a suffix denoting inflammation).

arterio-spasm. A contraction or spasm of an artery. / arterio / spasmos (G. seizure, spasm).

arthr-... **arthri-**... **arthro-**... Greek combining forms, from *arthron* (joint), referring to a *joint, articulation.*

arthro-centesis. Surgical puncture of a joint. / arthron / kentesis (G. a puncture).

-articul- . . . A combining form, from the Latin *articulatio* (articulation), referring to *joints.*

articul-ar. Pertaining to, or involving, an articulation or joint. / articul (joint) / ar (a suffix used to form adjectives).

articul-ator. A joint-like device used for holding casts of the jaws. / articul / ator (a suffix indicating an agent, that which).

-ary . . . An adjective-forming suffix, from the Latin *-arius,* meaning *pertaining to, connected with.*

heredit-ary. Derived from one's ancestors. / hereditas (L. inheritance) / ary.

-ary . . . A noun-forming suffix, from the Latin *-arius,* denoting *a person practicing a particular profession or trade, a thing used for a specified purpose.*

apothec-ary. A pharmacist; druggist. / apotheca (L. storehouse) / ary.

as- . . . A prefix having the same uses as the Latin *ad (to, toward, near, together),* but used instead of *ad* before the letter *s.*

as-simil-ation. The transformation of digested food into living matter. / ad (to) / similare (L. make similar) / ation (a noun-forming suffix indicating an *action*).

asc- . . . **asco-** . . . Greek combining forms, from *askos* (bag, bladder), referring to *a sac, bladder, bag.*

asco-mycete. One of a class of fungi reproducing from spores developed in a saclike structure. / askos / mykes (G. a fungus), genit. *myketos.*

-aster- . . . **asteri-** . . . Greek combining forms, from *aster* (star), denoting a relationship to *a star or a starlike structure.*

aster-oid. Shaped like a star. / aster / eides (G. having the form of).

astro- ... A Greek combining form, from *astron* (a star), referring to *a star, star-shaped structure.*

astro-cyte. A star-shaped cell of the nervous system. / astron / kytos (G. a cell).

at- ... A prefix having the same uses as the Latin *ad (to, toward, near, together),* but used instead of *ad* before the letter *t.*

at-tract-ion. A drawing together. / ad (to, together) / trahere, past participle *tractus* (draw) / ion (a noun-forming suffix indicating an *action*).

-ate ... 1. An adjective-forming suffix, from the Latin *-atus,* meaning *characterized by, shaped like.* 2. A verb-forming suffix meaning *become, produce, treat with.* 3. A noun-forming suffix denoting *office, agency, function, object or result of an action.*

umbilic-ate. Resembling a navel. / umbilicus (L. navel) / ate.

proli-fer-ate. To grow rapidly. / proles, genit. prolis (L. offspring) / ferre (L. to bear) / ate.

diplom-ate. The holder of a diploma. / diploma (G. a paper folded double) / ate.

-ation ... A noun-forming suffix, from the Latin *-ation, a process, action, condition.*

agglutin-ation. The clumping together of bacteria, blood cells, etc. / agglutinare (L. to glue together), past participle *agglutinatus* / ation.

atmo- ... A Greek combining form, from *atmos* (vapor), meaning *vapor, gas, air.*

atmo-sphere. The gaseous layer surrounding the earth. / atmos / sphaira (G. sphere).

atri-...   atrio-...   Combining forms, based on the Greek *atrion* (chamber), referring to an *auricle* or *atrium*.

atrio-megal-y. Enlargement of an atrium, especially of the heart. / atrio (atrium, chamber) / megas (G. big) / y (suffix denoting condition).

atri-al. Pertaining to an atrium. / atri / al (a suffix meaning *pertaining to*).

audi-...   audio-...   Latin combining forms, from *audire* (to hear), referring to *hearing*.

aud-ile. Pertaining to hearing. / audire / ile (a suffix meaning *having to do with*).

auricul-...   auriculo-...   Combining forms, derived from the Latin *auricula*, diminutive of *auris* (ear), denoting a relationship to the *ear*.

sub-auricul-ar. Situated below the ear. / sub (a Latin prefix meaning *beneath*) / auricula (ear) / ar (a Latin adjective-forming suffix).

aut-...   auto-...   Greek combining forms, from *autos* (self), meaning *self, own, oneself*.

aut-ops-y. An examination, with the aid of dissection, of a dead body, as in order to discover the cause of death. / autos / opsis (G. a sight or seeing) y (a noun-forming suffix indicating an *action*). *Note:* the semantic substance of "autopsy" is "a seeing with one's own eyes."

aux-...   auxi-...   auxo-...   Greek combining forms, from *auxein* (increase), meaning *increase, growth, stimulation*.

auxi-lyt-ic. Increasing the lytic or dissolving effect. / auxein / lytikos (G. loosing) / ic (an adjective-forming suffix).

avi-...   A Latin combining form, from *avis* (bird), referring to *birds*.

avi-culture. The rearing and care of birds. / avis / cultura (L. culture).

axi-... **axio-**... Combining forms from the Latin *axis* (an axle or axis), referring to an *axis*.

axi-fug-al. Moving away from an axis. / axi (axis) / fugere (L. flee) / al (an adjective-forming suffix).

axio-bucc-al. Pertaining to the axial and buccal walls of a tooth cavity. / axio / bucca (L. cheek) / al (an adjective-forming suffix).

-axill-... **-axillary**... **axillo-**... Combining forms, derived from the Latin *axilla* (armpit), referring to the *armpit* or *axilla*.

axill-ary. Pertaining to, or involving, the armpit. / axill (armpit) / ary (a suffix meaning *pertaining to*).

axillo-thoracic. Pertaining to, or involving, the armpit and the wall of the chest. / axillo / *thorax*, genit. *thorakos* (the chest). *Note: thorax* has the same form in Latin and in Greek.

azo-... A Greek combining form, from *a* (not) and *zoe* (life), referring to *nitrogen* (which does not support life).

azot-em-ia. An abnormal accumulation of nitrogen compounds in the blood. / azote (a former name for *nitrogen*) / haima (G. blood) / ia (a noun-forming suffix used in names of *disorders*).

B

bacill-... bacilli-... bacillo-... Combining forms, derived from the Latin *bacillus* (small rod or stick), referring to *bacilli* or *bacteria*.

bacill-emia. The presence of bacilli in the blood stream. / bacill (bacilli) / haima (G. blood). *Note:* the suffix *emia* denotes a condition of the blood, usually abnormal.

bacillo-phobia. An abnormal fear of bacilli or bacteria. / bacillo / phobos (G. fear).

bacter-... bacteri-... bacterio-... Combining forms from the Greek *bakterion* (a small rod), referring to *bacteria, bacilli*.

bacter-em-ia. The presence of bacteria in the blood. / bacter (bacteria) / haima (G. blood) / ia (a noun-forming suffix used in naming disorders).

bacteri-cid-al. Destructive to bacteria. / bacteri / caedere (L. to kill) / al (an adjective-forming suffix).

ballist-... ballisto-... Greek combining forms, from *ballein* (to throw), referring to *missiles, projectiles*.

ballisto-phob-ia. Abnormal fear of missiles. / ballein / phobos (G. fear) / ia (a noun-forming suffix denoting a *disorder*).

-bar-... baro-... Greek combining forms, from *baros* (weight), referring to *weight, pressure*.

18

baro-trauma. An injury caused by pressure or weight. / baros / trauma (G. injury).

batho-...   **bathy-**...   Greek combining forms, from *bathos* (depth) and *bathys* (deep), meaning *depth, deep.*

bathy-metr-y. The measurement of the depth range of marine life. / bathys / metron (G. measure) / y (a noun-forming suffix denoting an *action*).

bi-...   **bis-**...   Latin prefixes, from *bis* (twice), meaning *two, twice, double.*

bi-nom-ial. Designated by two names. / bis (L. twice) / nomen (L. name) / ial (an adjective-forming suffix denoting a *characteristic*).

biblio-...   A Greek combining form, from *biblion* (book), referring to a *book or books.*

biblio-pegy. The art or craft of bookbinding. / biblion / pegnynai (G. to bind).

biblio-graphy. A list of literary works of a given author or on a given subject. / biblion / graphia (writing), from *graphein* (G. to write).

bili-...   A combining form, derived from the Latin *bilis* (bile), indicating a relationship to *gall* or *bile.*

bili-ary. Pertaining to bile. / bili (bile) / ary (an adjective-forming suffix meaning *pertaining to*).

bili-rubin. A reddish bile pigment. / bili / ruber (L. red).

bio-...   A Greek combining form, from *bios* (life), meaning *life, living, involving living matter.*

bio-psy. The removal and examination of living tissue. / bios / opsis (G. a sight).

-blast-...   **blasto-**...   Combining forms, derived from the

Greek *blastos* (a bud), denoting a reference to an *embryonic stage, formative element, bud, germ.*

blast-oma. A tumor originating from embryonal cells. / blastos (formative element) / oma (G. a tumor).

blephar-... blepharo-... Greek combining forms, from *blepharon* (eyelid), referring to the *eyelid.*

blepharo-ptosis. A drooping of an eyelid. / blepharon / ptosis (G. a falling).

-bleps-... -blepsia... -blepsy... Greek combining forms, from *blepsis* (sight), referring to *sight, vision.*

mono-bleps-ia. The presence of normal vision in one eye only. / monos (G. one) / blepsis / ia (a noun-forming suffix used in names of *disorders*).

bov-... A Latin combining form, from *bos* (the ox), genit. *bovis,* referring to the *ox, cow, cattle.*

bov-ine. Derived from an ox or a cow; oxlike. / bovis / ine (a suffix meaning *having the nature of*).

brachi-... brachio-... Combining forms, from the Greek *brachion* (arm), referring to the *arm* or *upper extremity.*

brachi-algia. Pain in an arm. / brachi (arm) / algos (G. pain). *Note:* the suffix *ia* forms nouns indicating an abnormal condition.

brachio-cephalic. Pertaining to the arm and the head. / brachio / kephale (G. the head). *Note:* the suffix *ic* means *pertaining to.*

brachy-... A Greek prefix, from *brachys* (short), meaning *short, shortness.*

brachy-gnath-ia. The condition of having a short jaw. / brachys / gnathos (G. jaw) / ia (a noun-forming suffix denoting a *condition*).

brady- . . . A Greek prefix, from *bradys* (slow), meaning *slow, dull.*

brady-lex-ia. Abnormal slowness in reading. / bradys / lexis (G. speech, utterance) / ia (a noun-forming suffix indicating a *disorder*).

brom- . . . **bromo-** . . . Greek combining forms, from *bromos* (stench), meaning *malodorous, stench, rank odor.*

brom-hidrosis. Malodorous perspiration. / bromos / hidrosis (G. sweating).

-bronch- . . . **bronchi-** . . . **broncho-** . . . Combining forms, derived from the Greek *bronchos* (windpipe), referring to *bronchi* or a *bronchus.*

bronch-aden-itis. Inflammation of bronchial lymph nodes. / bronchos / aden (G. gland) / itis (a suffix denoting inflammation). *Note:* the ancient observers regarded the lymph nodes as glands.

bronchiol- . . . A combining form, derived from the Latin *bronchiolus* (a fine air passage), referring to a *bronchiole* or *bronchioles.*

bronchiol-ectasis. An abnormal dilatation of bronchioles. / bronchiolus (a bronchiole) / ektasis (G. extension, dilatation).

brux- . . . **bruxo-** . . . Greek combining forms, from *bryxis* (a gnashing) and *brykein* (to gnash), meaning *gnash, grind, gnaw.*

bruxo-mania. A neurotic gnashing of the teeth. / bryxis / mania (G. madness).

bucc- . . . **bucco-** . . . Combining forms, derived from the Latin *bucca* (cheek), denoting a reference to the *cheek* or *side of the face.*

bucco-lingu-al. Pertaining to the cheek and the tongue. / bucca (cheek) / lingua (L. tongue) / al (a Latin adjective-forming suffix meaning *pertaining to*).

burs- ... **burso-** ... Combining forms, derived from the Latin *bursa* (a pouch), referring to a *bursa, a sac filled with fluid.*

burs-ectom-y. The surgical removal of a bursa. / bursa / ektome (G. a cutting out) / y (a noun-forming suffix).

C

cac-... caco-... Combining forms, derived from the Greek *kakos* (bad), meaning *ill, deformed, bad, mean.*

cac-hexia. General bad health associated with malnutrition. / cac (bad) / echein (G. be).

caco-geusia. A sensation of bad taste. / caco / geusis (G. taste). *Note:* the suffix *ia* denotes a *condition.*

-calc-... calci-... calco-... Combining forms, derived from the Latin *calx,* genit. *calcis* (lime), denoting a relationship to *calcium, lime, chalk.*

hyper-calc-em-ia. The presence of too much calcium in the blood. / hyper (G. in excess) / calcis / haima (G. blood) / ia (a noun-forming suffix used in names of *disorders*).

calcane-... calcaneo-... Latin combining forms, from *calx* (heel), referring to the *calcaneus, heel bone.*

calcane-odyn-ia. Pain in the heel. / calx, genit. calcis / odyne (G. pain) / ia (a Latin noun-forming suffix used in names of *disorders, diseases*).

cali-... calli-... callo-... Greek combining forms, from *kallos* (beauty), meaning *beautiful, beauty.*

callo-mania. A mental disorder characterized by delusions of beauty. / kallos / mania (G. madness).

23

calor- . . .   **calori-** . . .   Latin combining forms, from *calor* (heat),
meaning *heat*.

calori-facient. Producing heat. / calor / facientis, present participle of facere (making).

canth- . . .   **cantho-** . . .   Combining forms, derived from the
Greek *kanthos* (the corner of the eye), referring to the *canthus*
or the *angle between the eyelids*.

cantho-plasty. A plastic operation on a canthus. / kanthos / plassein (G. to form).

capsul- . . .   **capsulo-** . . .   Combining forms, derived from the
Latin *capsula* (box), referring to a *capsule, box, case*.

capsul-ation. The formation of a capsule. / capsula / ation (a
Latin suffix used to form nouns denoting *a process*).

-carb- . . .   **carbo-** . . .   **carbon-** . . .   **carbono-** . . .   Combining forms, derived from the Latin *carbo* (coal), referring to
carbon, carbon dioxide, coal.

carb-ide. A compound of carbon and another substance. / carbo
/ ide (a suffix used in naming chemical compounds, usually those
consisting of two elements).

carbono-metry. The measurement of carbon dioxide. / carbo /
metron (G. measure) / y (a noun-forming suffix).

carbohydr- . . .   **carbohydrat-** . . .   **carbohydro-** . . .   Combining forms, derived from the Greek *hydor* (water) and the Latin
carbo (coal), referring to *carbohydrates*, a class of compounds
comprising the *sugars, starches*, and *celluloses*.

carbohydr-ase. An enzyme which splits carbohydrates. / carbo
(coal, carbon) / hydor (water) / ase (a Latin suffix used to form
names of *enzymes*).

carcin- . . .   **carcino-** . . .   Combining forms, derived from the
Greek *karkinos* (crab), referring to *cancer, carcinoma, malig-
nancy*.

carcino-genic. Producing or causing the formation of cancer. / karkinos / gignesthai (G. become) / ic (an adjective-forming suffix).

carcin-...   carcino-...   carcinomat-...   carcinomato-... Combining forms, derived from the Greek *karkinoma* (cancer), referring to *cancer, carcinoma.*

carcinomat-osis. The presence of multiple carcinomas. / karkinoma / osis (a Greek suffix indicating a *condition, disorder, disease*).

cardi-...   cardio-...   Greek combining forms, from *kardia* (heart), meaning *heart, cardiac sphincter of stomach.*

cardi-ectasis. Abnormal dilatation of the heart. / kardia / ektasis (G. dilatation).

-carpic...   carpo-...   -carpous...   Greek combining forms, from *karpos* (fruit), referring to *fruit, seeds.*

carpo-phag-ous. Subsisting mainly on fruit. / karpos / phagein (G. eat) / ous (an adjective-forming suffix meaning *characterized by*).

cata-...   A combining form, derived from the Greek *kata* (down), meaning *down, downward, low, inferior, under, along with.*

cata-basis. The decline of a disease. / kata (down) / bainein (G. to go).

caud-...   cauda-...   caudo-...   Latin combining forms, from *cauda* (tail), referring to a *tail or a taillike appendage.*

caud-ad. Toward the tail. / cauda / ad (a suffix meaning *toward*).

caud-ate. Having a tail or a taillike appendage. / cauda / ate (an adjective-forming suffix meaning *marked by, having*).

cava-...   cavi-...   cavit-...   cavo-...   Combining forms, derived from the Latin *cavitas* (a hollow), designating a reference to a *hollow space, cavity.*

cava-scope. An instrument used to examine cavities. / cavitas (hollow) / skopein (G. to look at, examine).

-cele ...   A Greek combining form, from *kele* (tumor), referring to a *hernia, tumor, swelling.*

adipo-cele. A hernia containing fat. / adeps, adipis (L. fat) / kele.

celi- ...   celio- ...   Combining forms referring to the *abdomen,* derived from the Greek *koilia,* the belly.

celi-alg-ia. Pain in the abdomen. / celi / algos (G. pain) / ia (a suffix used to form nouns).

celio-centesis. A surgical puncture of the abdominal wall. / celi / o (a word-joining particle) / kentesis (G. a puncture).

-cell- ...   celli- ...   cello- ...   cellu- ...   cellul- ...   celluli- ...   cellulo- ...   Combining forms, derived from the Latin *cella* (cell, compartment) and *cellula* (small cell), denoting a reference to a *cell, compartment, chamber, enclosure.*

celli-col-ous. Living within cells, as certain parasites. / cella (cell) / colere (L. to inhabit) / ous (a Latin adjective-forming suffix).

celluli-cid-al. Destructive to cells; killing cells. / cellula (small cell) / caedere (L. to kill) / al (a Latin adjective-forming suffix).

cen- ...   ceno- ...   Greek combining forms, from kainos (new), meaning *new, fresh, recent.*

ceno-phob-ia. An aversion for new things. / kainos / phobos (G. fear) / ia (a noun-forming suffix used in names of *disorders*).

cent- ...   centi- ...   Latin combining forms, from *centum* (hundred), meaning *hundred, hundredth, hundredfold.*

centi-grade. Divided into 100 gradations. / centum / gradus (L. step, degree).

-centesis ... A Greek terminal combining form, from *kentesis* (puncture), meaning *perforation, puncture, tapping.*

thoraco-centesis. A surgical puncture of the chest wall. / thorax, genit. thorakos (G. chest) / kentesis.

-centr- ... **centri-** ... **centro-** ... Combining forms, derived from the Latin *centrum* (center), referring to a *center, middle point, collection of nerve cells.*

centri-fug-al. Moving away from a center. / centrum (center) / fugere (L. to flee) / al (a Latin adjective-forming suffix meaning *characterized by*).

cephal- ... **cephalo-** ... Greek combining forms, from *kephale* (head), referring to the *head.*

cephal-alg-ia. Pain in the head. / kephale / algos (G. pain) / ia (a Latin noun-forming suffix used in names of *diseases*).

cept- ... **cepti-** ... **cepto-** ... Latin combining forms, from *receptus* (received), past participle of *recipere* (receive), meaning *receive, take, accept.*

extero-cept-ive. Receiving stimuli from the external environment. / externus (L. outward) / receptus, ceptus / ive (an adjective-forming suffix meaning *having the quality of*).

cer- ... **cera-** ... **cero-** ... Latin combining forms, from *cera* (wax), meaning *wax.*

cer-aceous. Waxlike. / cera / aceous (a suffix meaning *of the nature of*).

-cerebell- ... **cerebelli-** ... **cerebello-** ... Combining forms, derived from the Latin *cerebellum* (little brain), referring to the *cerebellum.*

cerebelli-fug-al. Moving away from the cerebellum. / cerebellum / fugere (L. to flee) / al (a Latin adjective-forming suffix meaning *characterized by*).

cerebr- ... **cerebri-** ... **cerebro-** ... Combining forms, derived from the Latin *cerebrum* (the upper anterior part of the brain), referring to the *cerebrum.*

cerebro-spinal. Pertaining to the brain and the spinal cord. / cerebrum / spina (L. the spine) / al (a Latin adjective-forming suffix meaning *pertaining to*).

cervic- ... **cervico-** ... Latin combining forms, from *cervix,* genit. *cervicis* (neck), referring to the *neck, cervix.*

cervic-ec-tom-y. The excision of the cervix of the uterus. / cervicis / ek (G. out) / tome (G. a cutting) / y (a suffix indicating an *action*).

chaet- ... **chaeti-** ... **chaeto-** ... Greek combining forms, from *chaite* (hair), referring to *hair, bristles.*

chaeti-ferous. Bearing or covered with bristles. / chaite / ferre (L. to bear) / ous (an adjective-forming suffix meaning *characterized by*).

chalc- ... **chalco-** ... Greek combining forms, from *chalkos* (copper), referring to *copper, brass.*

chalco-graphy. The art or practice of engraving on copper or brass plates. / chalkos / graphia (G. writing, from *graphein,* to write).

cheil- ... **cheilo-** ... Greek combining forms, from *cheilos* (lip), meaning *edge, margin, brim, lip.*

cheilo-plast-y. Plastic surgery on a lip. / cheilos / plastos (G. formed) / y (a suffix used in the formation of nouns indicating *action*).

cheir- ... **cheiro-** ... **chir-** ... **chiro-** ... Greek combining forms, from *cheir* (hand), referring to the *hand* or a *hand-like structure.*

cheiro-megal-y. Abnormal enlargement of a hand. / cheir / megas, megale (G. large) / y (a noun-forming suffix indicating a *condition*).

chem-... chemi-... chemico-... chemo-... Combining forms, derived from the Greek *kemeia* (transmutation), referring to *chemistry, chemical substance, chemical reaction.*

chemo-taxis. Movement of an organism in response to the influence of a chemical substance. / kemeia (transmutation, chemistry) / taxis (G. order, arrangement).

chlor-... chlori-... chloro-... Greek combining forms, from *chloros* (green), meaning *green, greenish.*

chloro-phyll. The green pigment of leaves. / chloros / phyllon (G. leaf).

chol-... chole-... cholo-... Combining forms, derived from the Greek *chole* (bile), meaning *biliary, bile.*

chol-agogue. A medicinal substance or any agent which stimulates the flow of bile. / chole (bile) / agein (G. to lead).

cholo-chrome. A biliary pigment. / cholo / chroma (G. color).

cholang-... cholangi-... cholangio-... Combining forms, derived from the Greek *chole* (bile) and *angeion* (vessel), indicating a relationship to a *bile duct.*

cholang-itis. Inflammation of a bile duct. / chol (bile) / ang (vessel) / itis (G. inflammation).

cholangi-ectasis. Abnormal dilatation of a bile duct. / cholangi / ectasis (G. dilatation).

cholecyst-... cholecysto-... Greek combining forms, from *chole* (bile) and *kystis* (bladder), meaning *gallbladder.*

chole-cyst-ek-tom-y. The surgical excision of the gallbladder. / chole / kystis / ek (G. out) / temnein (G. cut) / y (a suffix used to indicate an action).

choledoch-...   choledocho-...   Combining forms, derived from the Greek *chole* (bile) and *dochos* (containing), indicating a reference to the *common bile duct.*

chole-doch-ectomy. A surgical excision or removal of the common bile duct. / chole (bile) / dochos (containing) / ectomy (G. ek (out) and temnein (to cut)).

chole-docho-stomy. The surgical formation of an artificial opening in the common bile duct. / chole / docho / stomy (G. stoma, a mouth or opening) and y (a suffix forming nouns denoting a *condition*).

cholelith-...   cholelitho-...   Greek combining forms, from *chole* (bile) and *lithos* (stone), meaning *gallstone.*

chole-lith-iasis. The presence of gallstones in the biliary tract. / chole / lithos / iasis (a Greek suffix denoting a *process, diseased condition*).

-chondr-...   -chondro-...   Combining forms, derived from the Greek *chondros* (cartilage), denoting a reference to *cartilage, gristle.*

chondro-dys-troph-y. An abnormal growth or development of cartilage. / chondros / dys (abnormality) / trophe (G. food) / y (a noun-forming suffix denoting a *condition*).

chor-...   choro-...   Greek combining forms, from *choros* (region), referring to a *region, open area, country.*

choro-graphy. The art of describing or mapping a region. / choros / graphia (G. writing, from *graphein,* to write).

chord-...   chordo-...   Combining forms, derived from the Greek *chorde* (a cord), denoting a reference to a *cord, tract.*

chordo-tom-y. The surgical cutting of a nerve tract. / chorde (tract, cord) / temnein (G. to cut) / y (a noun-forming suffix denoting an *action*).

chore- ...   **choreo-** ...   Greek combining forms, from *choreia* (dance), referring to *dancing, dance.*

chore-ic. Pertaining to, or involving, chorea. / choreia / ic (an adjective-forming suffix meaning *pertaining to*).

chori- ...   **chorio-** ...   **choroid-** ...   **choroido-** ...   Combining forms, derived from the Greek *chorion* (the membrane surrounding the fetus), referring to the *chorion* (fetal membrane) and the *choroid* (the middle coat of the eyeball).

chorio-aden-oma. An adenoma of the chorion. / chorion / aden (G. a gland) / oma (a Greek suffix meaning *swelling, tumor*).

chorio-cele. A hernia of the eyeball in which the choroid is the protruding part. / chorion / kele (G. rupture, hernia).

-chrom- ...   **-chroma-** ...   **chromato-** ...   **chromo-** ...   Combining forms, derived from the Greek *chroma*, genit. *chromatos* (color), expressing a reference to *coloration, pigment, tint.*

chrom-affin. Staining readily with chromium dyes. / chrome (G. the metal chromium) / affinitas (G. union, affinity).

chron- ...   **chroni-** ...   **chrono-** ...   Greek combining forms, from *chronos* (time), referring to *time, duration.*

syn-chron-ous. Occurring simultaneously. / syn (G. together with) / chronos / ous (an adjective-forming suffix meaning *characterized by*).

chrys- ...   **chryso-** ...   Greek combining forms, from *chrysos* (gold), meaning *gold, golden, yellow.*

chrys-anthemum. A plant having showy flowers which bloom in late summer and fall. / chrysos / anthemon (G. flower).

chyl- ... **chyle-** ... **chyli-** ... **chylo-** ... Combining forms, derived from the Greek *chylos* (juice), referring to the *chyle*, the emulsion of fat globules in lymph formed in the small intestine during digestion.

chylo-rrhea. An excessive flow of chyle. / chylos (juice) / rhein (G. to flow). *Note:* the *r* in *chylorrhea* is doubled in accordance with the rule that when a Greek word (like *rhein*) beginning with an aspirated *r (rh)* is preceded by a prefix or other combining form ending in a short vowel, the letter *r* is repeated.

-cib- ... **ciba-** ... **cibo-** ... Latin combining forms, from *cibus* (food), meaning *nourishment, food.*

cibo-phob-ia. Fear of eating or of food. / cibus / phobos (G. fear) / ia (a Latin noun-forming suffix used in names of *disorders*).

cicatr- ... **cicatri-** ... **cicatrici-** ... **cicatrico-** ... Latin combining forms, from *cicatrix*, genit. *cicatricis* (a scar), referring to *scar tissue, scar.*

cicatr-ization. The formation of scar tissue in the process of healing. / cicatricis / ization (a noun-forming suffix denoting an *action, process*).

-cid- ... **-cide** ... Latin combining forms, from *caedere* (to kill), meaning *killing, killer, kill.*

spermato-cide. A substance capable of killing spermatozoa. / sperma, spermato (G. seed, sperm) / caedere.

cil- ... **-cili-** ... **cilio-** ... Latin combining forms, from *cilium* (eyelash), referring to an *eyelash, eyelid, ciliary body.*

super-cili-um. The structure above the eyelid; eyebrow. / super (L. above) / cilium / um (a neuter ending of nouns).

cine- ... **cinemat-** ... **cinemato-** ... **kine-** ... **kinemat-** ... **kinemato-** ... Greek combining forms, from *kinema*, genit. *kinematos* (motion), referring to *motion, movement.*

cine-photo-micro-graph-y. The making of a motion picture of minute objects. / kinema / phos, photos (G. light) / mikros (G. small) / graphein (G. to write) / y (a noun-forming suffix indicating a *process, action*).

cion-...   **ciono-**...   Greek combining forms, from *kion* (uvula), meaning *uvula*.

cion-itis. Inflammation of the uvula. / kion / itis (a suffix used to denote *inflammation*).

circum-...   A prefix, from the Latin *circum* (around), meaning *surrounding, around*.

circum-fer-ence. The outer margin of a round object; the boundary of any area. / circum (around) / ferre (L. to bear) / ence (a suffix forming nouns).

circum-corne-al. Surrounding the cornea, the transparent circular area in front of the eyeball. / circum / cornea (L. horny) / al (an adjective-forming suffix).

cirri-...   **cirro-**...   Latin combining forms, from *cirrus* (a curl), referring to *a curl or curl like structure*.

cirri-ped. A saltwater crustacean. / cirrus / pes (L. foot), genit. *pedis*.

-clas-...   **-clasis**...   Combining forms, derived from the Greek *klasis* (break), having reference to a *fracture, break, breakdown*.

histo-clast-ic. Capable of breaking down tissues. / histos (G. tissue) / klastos (G. broken) / ic (an adjective-forming suffix).

odonto-clasis. The fracture of a tooth. / *odous*, genit. *odontos* (G. a tooth) / klasis (break).

cleid-...   **cleido-**...   Combining forms, derived from the Greek *kleis*, genit. *kleidos* (key, bar, clavicle), referring to the *clavicle, collarbone*.

sterno-cleido-mast-oid. Pertaining to, or involving, the breast-bone, collarbone, and the mastoid process of the temporal bone. / sternon (breast, breastbone) / kleis, kleidos (collarbone) / mastos (G. breast, like a breast) / eidos (G. form, shape). *Note:* the suffix *oid* is used in the sense of *resembling.*

cleisto- ... A Greek combining form, from *kleistos* (closed), meaning *unopened, closed.*

cleisto-gamy. The condition of having self-pollinating, closed flowers. / kleistos / gamos (G. marriage).

clin- ... **clinic-** ... **clino-** ... Combining forms, derived from the Greek *kline* (bed) and *klinein* (to recline), referring to *lying, bedside, bed, horizontal posture.*

clin-ician. An expert in clinical or bedside medicine. / clin (bedside) / ician (a suffix indicating one skilled in a particular field).

clino-therap-y. Treatment of disease by rest in bed. / clino / therapeuein (G. take care of) / y (a suffix forming nouns).

co- ... A variant of the Latin prefix *com* (which see), used before *gn, h,* and *vowels.*

co-here. To stick together. / co (together) / haerere (L. to stick).

-cocc- ... **cocci-** ... **cocco-** ... Combining forms, derived from the Latin *coccus* (kernel), referring to *spherical micro-organisms.*

cocco-bacillus. A microorganism whose shape is midway between a coccus and a bacillus. / coccus or kokkos (G. kernel or berry) / bacillus (L. a small rod).

coccy- ... **coccyg-** ... **coccygo-** ... Combining forms, derived from the Greek *kokkyx* (the cuckoo, in allusion to its bill), genit. *kokkygos,* denoting the *coccyx.*

coccyg-odyn-ia. Pain in the coccyx or in the region of the coccyx. / kokkyx (coccyx) / odyne (G. pain) / ia (a Latin noun-forming suffix used in names of *diseases* and *disorders*).

coen-... coeno-... Greek combining forms, from *koinos* (common), meaning *common*.

coeno-cyte. A mass of protoplasm containing several nuclei. / koinos / kytos (G. a cell).

col-... A variant form of the Latin prefix *com* (which see), used before the letter *l*.

col-later-al. Running side by side with something specified. / col (together) / latus (a side), genit. *lateris* / al (an adjective-forming suffix meaning *having the characteristics of*).

-col-... coli-... colo-... colon-... Combining forms, derived from the Greek *kolon* (large bowel), referring to the *colon, large intestine*.

colo-enter-itis. Inflammation of the colon and small intestine. / kolon (large intestine, colon) / enteron (G. intestine, small intestine) / itis (a suffix used to indicate *inflammation*).

cole-... coleo-... Greek combining forms, from *koleos* (a sheath), meaning *vagina*.

cole-itis. Inflammation of the vagina. / koleos / itis (a suffix used to denote *inflammation*).

-colous A Latin terminal combining form, from *colere* (inhabit), meaning *growing, living, inhabiting*.

terri-colous. Living in or on the ground. / terra (L. earth) / colere / ous (an adjective-forming suffix denoting a *characteristic*).

colp-... colpi-... colpo-... Greek combining forms, from *kolpos* (womb), meaning *vagina, womb, hollow*.

colpo-scope. An instrument for examining the vagina. / kolpos / scope (a suffix denoting an instrument for viewing, from the Greek *skopein*, to watch).

com-... A Latin prefix, from *cum* (with), meaning *with, together, in association. Note: com* changes to *co* before *gn*, *h*, and *vowels;* to *col* before *l;* to *con* before *c, d, f, g, j, n, q, s, t, v;* to *cor* before *r; com* is used before *b, m, p.*

com-pat-ible. Capable of existing together. / com / pati (L. to feel) / ible (a suffix meaning *able to*).

con- ... A variant form of the Latin prefix *com* (which see), used before the letters *c, d, f, g, j, n, q, s, t, v.*

con-cres-ence. A growing together. / con (together) / crescere (L. to grow) / ence (a noun-forming suffix denoting an *action*).

con- ...   **cono-** ...   Greek combining forms, from *konos* (cone), meaning *cone, wedge.*

con-odont. Having wedge-shaped teeth. / konos / odon (G. tooth), genit. *odontos.*

-condyl- ...   **condylo-** ...   Combining forms, derived from the Greek *kondylos* (knuckle), referring to a *condyle, rounded projection.*

condyl-ectom-y. Excision or cutting out of a condyle. / kondylos (condyle) / ektome (G. a cutting out) / y (a Latin noun-forming suffix denoting an *action* or *result of an action*).

contra- ...   A prefix, derived from the Latin *contra* (against), meaning *opposite, contrary, opposed, against.*

contra-cept-ive. A medicinal substance, or any agent, which prevents conception or impregnation. / contra (opposing) / conceptio (L. conception) / ive (an adjective-forming suffix).

contra-dict. To assert the opposite, as of a statement. / contra (opposite) / dicere (L. to speak).

copr- ...   **copro-** ...   Greek combining forms, from *kopros* (dung), meaning *feces, excrement, dung, stool.*

copro-lith. A concentration or "stone" composed of fecal matter. / kopros / lithos (G. stone).

-cor- . . .   core- . . .   coreo- . . .   cori- . . .   coro- . . .   Greek combining forms, from *kore* (pupil), meaning *pupil of the eye.*

cor-ec-top-ia. Displacement of the pupil from the normal position. / kore / ek (G. out) / topos (G. place) / ia (a noun-forming suffix used in names of *disorders*).

cor- . . .   A variant form of the Latin prefix *com* (which see), used before the letter *r*.

cor-respond. To conform; be in agreement. / cor (together) / respondere (L. to answer).

corti- . . .   cortic- . . .   cortici- . . .   cortico- . . .   Combining forms, derived from the Latin *cortex*, genit. *corticis* (rind), referring to a *cortex, outer layer.*

cortico-trop-ic. Influencing the cortex, as of the brain. / corticis (of the cortex) / trope (G. a turning) / ic (a Latin adjective-forming suffix).

-cost- . . .   costi- . . .   costo- . . .   Latin combining forms, from *costa* (rib), meaning *rib, riblike ridge.*

cost-alg-ia. Pain in a rib. / costa / algos (G. pain) / ia (a noun-forming suffix used in names of *disorders*).

counter- . . .   A Latin prefix, from *contra* (against), meaning *opposite, against, contrary to.*

counter-irritation. An irritation which opposes another irritation. / contra / irritatio (L. irritation).

cox- . . .   coxi- . . .   coxo- . . .   Latin combining forms, from *coxa* (hip), referring to the *hip joint, hip.*

cox-arthro-path-y. Disease of the hip joint. / coxa / arthron (G. joint) / pathos (G. disease) / y (a suffix denoting a *condition*).

-cracy . . .   A Greek combining form, from *kratos* (rule), referring to *a designated type of government, rule by.*

theo-cracy. Government by those who claim to rule by divine authority. / theos (G. god) / kratia, kratos.

-crani-...   cranio-...   Combining forms, derived from the Latin *cranium* (skull), referring to the *cranium, skull.*

cranio-logy. The study of skulls. / cranium (skull) / logy (a suffix denoting a *study, science*).

-cric-...   crico-...   cricoid-...   Combining forms, derived from the Greek *krikos* (a ring), referring to the *cricoid cartilage.*

cricoid-ectom-y. Excision of the cricoid cartilage. / krikos (ring, cricoid cartilage) / ektome (G. a cutting out) / y (a noun-forming suffix denoting an *action* or the *result of an action*).

-crin-...   crino-...   Greek combining forms, from *krinein* (separate, secrete), referring to *secretion.*

endo-crino-logy. The science of endocrine glands and their secretions. / endon (G. within) / krinein / logy (science of, from *logos,* G. word, study).

cruc-...   cruci-...   Latin combining forms, from *crux* (cross), genit. *crucis,* referring to *a cross or crosslike structure.*

cruci-ate. Shaped like a cross. / crucis / ate (an adjective-forming suffix meaning *shaped like*).

crur-...   cruri-...   cruro-...   Latin combining forms, from *crus,* genit. *cruris* (a leg), referring to a *leg, leglike structure, shin.*

cruro-femor-al. Pertaining to the leg and thigh. / crus, cruris / femur (L. thigh) / al (a Latin adjective-forming suffix meaning *pertaining to*).

cry-...   cryo-...   Combining forms, derived from the Greek *kryos* (cold), denoting *cold, frost, freezing.*

cry-alges-ia. Pain caused by cold. / kryos (cold) / algesis (G. feeling of pain) / ia (a Latin noun-forming suffix used in names of *diseases* and *disorders*).

crypt-... **crypto-**... Greek combining forms, from *kryptos* (hidden), meaning *hidden, concealed, secret.*

crypt-esthes-ia. Subconscious perception. / kryptos (hidden) / aisthesis (G. sensation) / ia (a Latin noun-forming suffix used in names of disorders).

crystall-... **crystallo-**... Greek combining forms, from *crystallos* (crystal), referring to *a crystal.*

cystall-ize. To form crystals. / krystallos / ize (a verb-forming suffix meaning *cause to be, become*).

cten-... **cteno-**... Greek combining forms, from *kteis* (a comb), genit. *ktenos,* referring to *a comb or comblike structure.*

cten-oid. Having projections resembling the teeth of a comb. / ktenos / eides (G. having the shape or form of).

cupr-... **cupri-**... **cupro-**... Latin combining forms, from *cuprum* (copper), referring to *copper.*

cupri-fer-ous. Bearing or containing copper. / cuprum / ferre (L. to bear) / ous (an adjective-forming suffix meaning *having*).

-cut-... **cuti-**... Latin combining forms, from *cutis* (skin), meaning *skin, membrane.*

cuti-sect-or. An instrument for cutting off thin layers of skin. / cutis / sectus, past participle of *secare* (to cut) / or (a suffix denoting a person or thing performing a specified function).

cutane-... A Latin combining form, from *cutaneus* (pertaining to skin), meaning *skin, of the skin.*

sub-cutane-ous. Under the skin. / sub (beneath) / cutaneus / ous (an adjective-forming suffix).

cuticul- ...   A Latin combining form, from *cuticula* ("little skin"), a diminutive of *cutis* (skin), referring to *skin, covering membrane*.

cuticul-ar-ization. The formation of new skin, as on a wound. / cuticula / ar (an adjective-forming suffix meaning *like*) / ization (a noun-forming suffix denoting a *process*).

-cy ...   A noun-forming suffix, from the Latin *-cia,* denoting *a condition, status, fact of being.*

idio-cy. The condition of being an idiot. / idiotes (G. ignorant person) / cy.

cyan- ...   **cyani-** ...   **cyano-** ...   Combining forms, derived from the Greek *kyanos* (blue), denoting a reference to the color *blue* and to *cyanic acid.*

cyano-phil. Fond of the color blue; staining readily with blue dyes. / kyanos (blue) / philein (G. to love).

cyan-ate. A salt of cyanic acid. / kyanos / ate (a suffix used to designate *salts* and *esters*).

cycl- ...   **cycli-** ...   **cyclo-** ...   Combining forms, derived from the Greek *kyklos* (circle), carrying the concept of *circle, rotation, ciliary body, round.*

cyclo-phor-ia. A tendency of the eyeball to roll outward or inward. / kyklos (circle) / phorein (G. bear, move) / ia (a Latin noun-forming suffix used in names of disorders).

cyclo-pleg-ia. Paralysis of the ciliary muscle or body./kyklos (circle, ciliary body) / plege (G. a stroke) / ia (a Latin noun-forming suffix used in names of *diseases* and *disorders*).

cyes- ...   **cyesi-** ...   **cyesio-** ...   **cyeso-** ...   Greek combining forms, from *kyesis* (gestation), referring to *pregnancy, gestation, conception.*

cyes-edema. Swelling associated with pregnancy. / kyesis / oidema (G. swelling).

cylindr- ... **cylindri-** ... **cylindro-** ... Combining forms, derived from the Greek *kylindros* (a roller), referring to a *cylinder, column, roller.*

cylindri-form. Shaped like a cylinder. / kylindros (roller) / forma (L. shape).

cyn- ... **cyni-** ... **cyno-** ... Combining forms, derived from the Greek *kyon*, genit. *kynos* (dog), referring to dogs.

cyno-phob-ia. Abnormal fear of dogs. / kyon (dog) / phobos (G. fear) / ia (a Latin noun-forming suffix used in names of disorders)

cyprid- ... **cyprido-** ... Greek combining forms, from *Kypris*, genit. *Kypridos* (Venus or Aphrodite), referring to *lewdness, venereal disease. Note:* The allusion is to *Kypros*, the Greek name of Cyprus, where the ancients worshipped Aphrodite, the goddess of love.

cyprido-phob-ia. Abnormal fear of venereal disease. / Kypridos / phobos (G. fear) / ia (a noun-forming suffix used in names of *disorders*).

-cyst- ... **cysti-** ... **cystido-** ... **cysto-** ... Combining forms, derived from the Greek *kystis* (a sac), referring to a *cyst, urinary bladder, gallbladder.*

poly-cyst-ic. Containing several cysts. / polys (G. many) / kystis (sac) / ic (an adjective-forming suffix).

cysto-lith. A calculus or "stone" of the urinary bladder. / kystis / lithos (G. stone).

cyt- ... **-cyte** ... **-cyti-** ... **cyto-** ... Combining forms, derived from the Greek *kytos* (a hollow vessel), referring to a *cell, vessel, container, cover.*

erythro-cyte. A red blood cell. / erythros (G. red) / kytos (cell).

cyto-plasm. The protoplasm of a cell, as opposed to the protoplasm of the nucleus. / kytos / plasma (G. something molded).

D

-dacry- . . .   **dacryo-** . . .   Greek combining forms, from *dakry-on* (a tear), referring to *tears, lacrimal apparatus.*

dacry-ops. A watery condition of the eyes; an excessive discharge of tears. / dakryon / ops (G. the eye).

dacryaden- . . .   **dacryoaden-** . . .   **dacryoadeno-** . . .   Greek combining forms, from *dakryon* (a tear) and *aden* (gland), referring to the *lacrimal gland.*

dacryo-aden-itis. Inflammation of a lacrimal gland. / dakryon / aden / itis (a noun-forming suffix meaning *inflammation*).

dacryocyst- . . .   **dacryocysti-** . . .   **dacryocysto-** . . .   Greek combining forms, from *dakryon* (a tear) and *kystis* (a sac), referring to a *lacrimal sac.*

dacryo-cyst-ectas-ia. Abnormal dilatation of a lacrimal sac. / dakryon / kystis / ektasis (G. distention, dilatation) / ia (a noun-forming suffix used in names of disorders).

-dactyl- . . .   **dactylo-** . . .   **dactylo-** . . .   Greek combining forms, from *daktylos* (finger), meaning *finger, toe, digit.*

dactylo-gryposis. A permanent flexion of a finger or toe. / daktylos / gryposis (G. a bending).

de- . . .   A Latin prefix, based on *de* (from), meaning *from, away from, down, off, reverse.*

de-capit-ate. To cut off the head of. / de / caput (L. head) / ate (a verb-forming suffix).

deca-...   A Greek combining form, from *deka* (ten), meaning *ten, tenfold.*

deca-meter. A measure of length equal to ten meters. / deka / metron (G. measure).

deci-...   A Latin prefix, from *decem* (ten), meaning *one tenth.*

deci-gram. One tenth part of a gram. / decem / gram, gramma (G. small weight).

deglutit-...   **deglutiti-**...   **-gluti-**...   Latin combining forms, from *deglutire* (to swallow), past participle *deglutitus,* referring to *swallowing.*

deglutit-odyn-ia. A condition in which swallowing causes pain. / deglutitus / odyne (G. pain) / ia (a noun-forming suffix denoting a *disorder*).

demi-...   A Latin prefix, from *dimidius* (half), meaning *half, intermediate.*

demi-facet. Half of a facet. / dimidius / facies (L. face).

demo-...   A Greek combining form, from *demos* (the people), referring to *people, population.*

demo-graphy. The science concerned with the distribution, density, etc., of populations. / demos / graphia (G. writing), from *graphein* (to write).

dendr-...   **dendri-**...   **dendro-**...   **-dendron**...   Greek combining forms, from *dendron* (tree), referring to *a tree, tree-like structure.*

dendr-ite. The branched process of a nerve cell. / dendron / ite (a noun-forming suffix used to denote *a structure of a certain kind*).

-dent- ...   **denti-** ...   **dento-** ...   Latin combining forms, from *dens* (tooth), genit. *dentis,* meaning *tooth, teeth.*

e-dent-ia. The condition of having no teeth; toothlessness. / e (a prefix meaning *without*) / dentis / ia (a noun-forming suffix used to denote a *disorder*).

-derm- ...   **derma-** ...   **dermat-** ...   **dermato-** ...   **dermo-** ...   Greek combining forms, from *derma* (skin), genit. *dermatos,* meaning *skin, derma, dermis.*

hypo-derm-ic. Pertaining to, or involving, the tissues under the skin. / hypo (beneath) / derma / ic (an adjective-forming suffix meaning *pertaining to*).

desm- ...   **desmio-** ...   **desmo-** ...   Greek combining forms, from *desmos* (band), meaning *ligament, band, bundle.*

desm-ectasis. Abnormal stretching of a ligament. / desmos / ektasis (G. a stretching, extension).

deuter- ...   **deutero-** ...   **deuto-** ...   Greek combining forms, from *deuteros* (second), meaning *second, secondary.*

deuter-an-op-ia. A form of color blindness marked by the inability to see green colors. / deuteros (second, in allusion to the fact that green is the second of the primary colors) / an (not, without) / opsis (G. vision) / ia (a noun-forming suffix used in names of *disorders*).

dextr- ...   **dextri-** ...   **dextro-** ...   Latin combining forms, from *dexter* (right), meaning *right, right side, on the right.*

dextr-aur-al. Hearing better with the right ear. / dexter / auris (L. ear) / al (an adjective-forming suffix meaning *characterized by*).

di- ...   A Greek prefix, from *dis* (twice), meaning *two, twice, double.*

di-cephal-us. A fetal monster having two heads. / dis / kephale

(G. head) / us (a suffix forming nouns meaning *one who has a specified characteristic*).

di-... dia-... Greek prefixes, from *dia* (through), meaning *through, across, apart, between.*

dia-pedesis. The passage of blood cells through the wall of a blood vessel. / dia / pedesis (G. a leaping, oozing).

di-... dif-... dis-... Latin prefixes conveying a variety of concepts, chiefly *separation* and *reversal. Note: di-* is used before *b, d, g, l, m, n, r, v; dif-* is used before *f.*

di-late. To make wider. / di (separation) / latus (L. wide).

-digit-... digiti-... digito-... Combining forms, derived from the Latin *digitus* (finger, toe), referring to a *finger, toe, digit.*

digiti-grade. Walking on the toes. / digitus (toe) / gradi (L. to walk).

dino-... A Greek combining form, from *deinos* (terrible), meaning *dreadful, terrible.*

dino-saur. An extinct reptile of the Mesozoic Era. / deinos / sauros (G. lizard).

dipl-... diplo-... Combining forms, derived from the Greek *diploos* (double), *meaning twice, double, twofold, twin.*

dipl-opia. Double vision. / diploos (double) / ops (G. eye) / ia (a Latin noun-forming suffix used in names of *disorders*).

disco-... A combining form, derived from the Latin *discus* or the Greek *diskos* (a disk), referring to an intervertebral *disk.*

disco-path-y. Disease of an intervertebral disk. / discus (disk) / pathos (G. disease) / y (a noun-forming suffix denoting a *condition*).

dist-... **disto-**...   Combining forms, derived from the Latin *distantia* (distance), meaning *farther, remote, distal.*

disto-bucc-al. Pertaining to the distal and buccal surfaces of a tooth. / distantia (distance) / bucca (L. cheek) / al (a Latin adjective-forming suffix).

dolicho-...   A Greek combining form, from *dolichos* (long), meaning *long, elongated.*

dolicho-cephal-ic. Having a long head. / dolichos / kephale (G. head) / ic (an adjective-forming suffix meaning *marked by*).

dorm-... **dormi-**... **dormo-**...   Latin combining forms, from *dormire* (to sleep), meaning *sleep, inactive, quiescent.*

ob-dormi-tion. Numbness of a part resulting from pressure on a nerve. / ob (upon) / dormire / tion (a noun-forming suffix denoting a *condition*).

dors-... **dorsi-**... **dorso**...   Combining forms, derived from the Latin *dorsum* (back), meaning *back, posterior, dorsum.*

dors-ad. Directed toward the back. / dors (back) / ad (L. toward).

dorso-later-al. Pertaining to the back and side. / dorso / *latus*, genit. *lateris* (L. side). *Note: al* is an adjective-forming suffix.

dos-... **dosi-**... **doso-**...   Combining forms, derived from the Greek *dosis* (a dose), referring to *dosage* or a *dose.*

micro-dos-age. Administration of minute doses. / mikros (G. small) / dosis (dose) / age (a noun-forming suffix indicating *amount*).

drepan-... **drepani-**... **drepano-**...   Greek combining forms, from *drepanon* (a sickle), meaning *semilunar, crescent, sickle.*

drepano-cyte. An abnormal red blood cell having the shape of a sickle. / drepanon / kytos (G. cell).

-drom-... **dromi-**... **dromo-**... Greek combining forms, from *dromos* (a running race), referring to *running, conduction.*

pro-drom-al. Premonitory; coming before something else. / pro (before) / dromos (a running), dramein (to run) / al (an adjective-forming suffix meaning *having the characteristics of*).

-duc-... **-duct-**... Latin combining forms, from *ducere* (to lead), meaning *lead, conduct, convey.*

ab-duc-ent. Moving away; abducting. / ab (away) / ducere / ent (an adjective-forming suffix).

duoden-... **duodeno-**... Combining forms, derived from the Latin *duodeni* (twelve each), referring to the *duodenum, first part of the small intestine. Note:* the "twelve each" in the preceding refers to the length of the structure, which is about twelve fingers' breadth.

duodeno-hepat-ic. Pertaining to the duodenum and the liver. / duodeni / *hepatos*, genit. of *hepar* (G. liver) / ic (a Latin adjective-forming suffix).

-dur-... **dura-**... Latin combining forms, from *durus* (hard), meaning *hard, firm.*

in-dur-ate. To become, or to cause to become, hard. / in (intensifier) / durus / ate (a Latin verb-forming suffix meaning *to become*).

-dynam-... **dynamo-**... Greek combining forms, from *dynamis* (power), meaning *power, force, strength.*

nucleo-dynam-ous. Pertaining to, or involving, nuclear power. / nucleus (L. nut, kernel) / dynamis / ous (an adjective-forming suffix meaning *pertaining to*).

dys- . . .   A prefix, derived from the Greek *dys* (bad, difficult), meaning *difficult, painful, hard, faulty, impaired, unlike.*

dys-peps-ia. Impaired digestion. / dys (impaired) / pepsis (G. digestion, cooking) / ia (a Latin noun-forming suffix used in names of *diseases* and *disorders*).

dys-pnea. Difficult breathing; shortness of breath. / dys (difficult) / pnoe (G. breathing).

E

e-... A prefix having the same meanings as *ex-* (which see) but used instead of *ex-* before a word or a combining form beginning with one of the following letters: *b, d, g, h, l, m, n, r, v.*

e-merg-ency. A sudden occurrence demanding immediate action. / e (out) / mergere (L. to dip) / ency (a Latin noun-forming suffix meaning a *state*).

ec-... A prefix having the same meanings as *ex-* (which see) but used instead of *ex-* before a word or a combining form beginning with the letter *c* or *s*.

ec-centr-ic. Not having the same center; off center. / ec (away from) / centrum (L. center) / ic (an adjective-forming suffix).

ec-... A prefix, from the Greek *ek* (out), meaning *out, out of, from.*

ec-chondr-oma. A tumor growing out of cartilage. / ek (out) / chondros (G. cartilage) / oma (G. tumor).

echo-... A Greek combining form, from *echo* (returned sound), meaning *imitation, repetition, mimicry.*

echo-lal-ia. Repetition by patient of words addressed to him. / echo / lalein (G. speak) / ia (a Latin noun-forming suffix used in names of *disorders*).

ecto-... A Greek prefix, from *ektos* (outside), meaning *outside, external, outer.*

ecto-zoon. A parasite living on the external surface of the host. / ektos / zoion (G. an animal).

-ectomize . . .   **-ectomy** . . .   Greek combining forms, from *ek* (out) and *temnein* (to cut), referring to a *cutting* or *excision*.

nephr-ec-tom-ize. To excise a kidney. / nephros (G. kidney) / ek (out) / temnein (cut) / ize (a verb-forming suffix).

ectro- . . .   A combining form, derived from the Greek *ektrosis* (miscarriage, abortion), meaning *congenital absence*.

ectro-dactyl-y. Congenital absence of a finger or toe. / ektrosis (congenital absence of) / daktylos (G. finger, toe) / y (a Latin noun-forming suffix indicating a *condition*).

-edem- . . .   **edema-** . . .   **edemat-** . . .   **edemato-** . . .   Greek combining forms, from *oidema* (a swelling), genit. *oidematos*, referring to a *swelling, tumor, edema*.

edemat-ization. The process of swelling or becoming swollen. / oidematos / ization (a noun-forming suffix denoting a *process*).

ef- . . .   A prefix having the same significance as *ex-* (which see) but used instead of *ex-* before a word or a combining form beginning with the letter *f*.

ef-femin-ate. Having the qualities or characteristics attributed to women. / ef (out) / femina (L. a woman) / ate (an adjective-forming suffix).

eid- . . .   **eido-** . . .   Greek combining forms, from *eidos* (form), meaning *form, shape, configuration*.

eido-log-y. The study of form. / eidos / logos (G. word, study) / y (a noun-forming suffix).

eid- . . .   **eido-** . . .   **-ode** . . .   **-oid** . . .   **-oidal** . . .   **-oidea** . . .   **-oidus** . . .   Greek combining forms, from *eidos* (form) and oeides (in the form of), meaning *like, resembling, having the form of*.

rhomb-oid-eus. A muscle of the back. / rhombos (G. a spinning top) / oeides (resembling) / eus (a noun-forming suffix used in *scientific names*). *Note:* the name of the muscle is an allusion to a rhombus, an equilateral parallelogram.

-eikon-... **icon-**... **icono-**...   Greek combining forms, from *eikon* (image), meaning *image, picture, illustration.*

anis-eikon-ia. Inequality of the images in the two eyes. / anisos (G. unequal) / eikon / ia (a Latin noun-forming suffix used in names of *disorders*).

elast-... **elasti-**... **elasto-**...   Combining forms, derived from the Greek *elastikos* (elastic), meaning *resilient, springy, elastic.*

elasto-lytic. Capable of dissolving elastic tissue. / elastikos (elastic) / lysis (G. a loosening) / ic (a Latin adjective-forming suffix).

electr-... **electro-**...   Combining forms, derived from the Greek *elektron* (amber), referring to *electricity. Note:* electricity was first noted and generated in amber, by friction.

electro-cardio-gram. A record of the electric currents produced by the action of the heart. / elektron / kardia (G. heart) / gramma (letter, writing).

em-...   A Latin prefix, used instead of *en* before *b, p,* and *m,* meaning *in, into, on.*

em-pye-ma. An accumulation of pus in a cavity of the body. / em / pyein (G. suppurate) / ma (a noun-forming suffix denoting the *result of an action*).

embol-... **emboli-**... **embolo-**...   Greek combining forms, from *embolos* (plug), referring to an *embolus, clot, plug.*

embol-ec-tom-y. The excision of an embolus. / embolos (plug, embolus) / ek (G. out) / temnein (cut) / y (a noun-forming suffix indicating an *action*).

embry-...   embryo-...   Greek combining forms, from *embryon* (embryo), referring to an *embryo*.

embryo-genesis. The development of an embryo. / embryon / genesis (G. origin, development).

-emia ...   hem-...   hema-...   hemat-...   hemato-... hemo-...   Combining forms, derived from the Greek *haima*, genit. *haimatos* (blood), indicating a relationship to *blood*.

hem-angi-oma. A tumor composed of young blood vessels. / haima (blood) / angeion (G. a vessel) / oma (G. a tumor).

hemat-ur-ia. The discharge of urine containing blood. / haimatos / ouron (G. urine) / ia (a noun-forming suffix).

en-...   A Latin prefix meaning *in, into, on.*

en-cephal-on. The brain tissue within the cranium. / en / kephale (G. head) / os (G. noun-forming suffix). *Note:* the *on* of *encephalon* is a modification of *os.*

encephal-...   encephali-...   encephalo-...   Combining forms, derived from the Greek *enkephalos* (brain), having a reference to the *brain* or *encephalon.*

encephal-itis. Inflammation of the brain. / en (in) / kephale (G. head) / itis (a suffix denoting *inflammation*).

end-...   endo-...   Greek combining forms, from *endon* (within), meaning *within, inside, inner.*

endo-crani-al. Situated within the cranium. / endon (within) / kranion (G. skull) / al (an adjective-forming suffix denoting a *characteristic*).

ent-...   ento-...   Greek combining forms, from *entos* (inside), meaning *inside, within, inner.*

ento-cele. An internal hernia. / entos (inside) / kele (G. a hernia, tumor).

-ent... 1. An adjective-forming suffix, from the Latin *-entis,* meaning *characterized by, having the quality of, performing the action of.* 2. A noun-forming suffix denoting *one who or that which performs a specified function.*

in-congru-ent. Not in agreement. / in (not) / congruere (L. to agree), present participle *congruence,* genitive *congruentis* / ent.

super-intend-ent. One who manages or directs. / super (L. over) / intendere (L. to stretch out for) / ent.

enter-...   enteri-...   entero-... Greek combining forms, from *enteron* (intestine), meaning *intestine.*

gastro-entero-log-y. The science of the stomach and intestine. / gaster (G. stomach) / enteron / logos (word, study) / y (a suffix denoting a *science*).

entom-...   entomo-... Greek combining forms, from *entomon* (insect), meaning *insect.*

en-tomo-phil-ous. Fond of insects. / en (G. in) / temnein (G. to cut) / philein (G. to love) / ous (an adjective-forming suffix).

eo-... Greek prefix, from *eos* (dawn), meaning *early, earliest.*

eo-hippus. A progenitor of the modern horse. / eos / hippos (G. horse).

-eous... An adjective-forming suffix, from the Latin *-eus,* meaning *like, of the nature of.*

vitr-eous. Pertaining to or resembling glass. / vitrum (L. glass) / eous.

ep-...   eph-...   epi-... Greek prefixes, from *epi* (on), meaning *on, upon, over, outside, beside.*

ep-hemeral. Lasting only a day. / epi / hemera (G. day) / al (an adjective-forming suffix).

equa-... equi-... Latin combining forms, from *aequus* (equal), meaning *equal, of the same quantity, intensity, etc.*

equi-later-al. Having equal sides. / aequus / latus, genit, lateris (L. the side) / al (a Latin adjective-forming suffix).

-er... A noun-forming suffix, from the Latin *-arius*, denoting *a person or thing performing a specified activity.*

lexico-graph-er. A person who writes a dictionary. / lexikon (G. a lexicon, dictionary) / graphein (G. to write) / er.

ereth-... erethi-... erethis-... erethiso-... Greek combining forms, from *erethizein* (arouse), meaning *stimulating, exciting, arousing, provoking.*

erethiso-phren-ia. Excessive mental excitability. / erethizein / phren (G. mind) / ia (a noun-forming suffix used in names of *disorders*).

erg-... ergas-... ergasi-... ergasio-... ergo-... Greek combining forms, from *ergon* and *ergasia* (work), referring to *work, labor, energy.*

ergasi-dermat-osis. An occupational dermatosis. / ergasia / derma, dermatos (G. skin) / osis (a suffix denoting a *disorder*).

erot-... eroti-... erotic-... erotico-... eroto-... Greek combining forms, from *eros* (love), genit. *erotos, erotikos* (lustful), meaning *sexual desire, sexual love, lust.*

eroto-phob-ia. Fear of, or aversion for, sexual love. / erotos / phobos (G. fear) / ia (a noun-forming suffix denoting a *disorder*).

erysi-... Greek prefix meaning *red.*

erysi-pelas. A skin disease marked by redness; red skin. / erysi (G. red) / pella (G. hide, skin).

eryth-... erythr-... erythro-... Greek combining forms, from *erythros* (red), meaning *red.*

erythro-cyte. A red blood cell. / erythros / kytos (G. cell).

es- ... A prefix having the same significance as *ex-* (which see) but used instead of *ex-* before a word or a combining form beginning with the letter *c* and before words borrowed from Old French.

es-cape. To slip away; break loose. / es (out of) / cappa (L. cloak, cape; i.e. leave one's cape behind).

-escence ... A noun-forming suffix, from the Latin *-escens*, indicating *a process, the act of becoming.*

bio-lumin-escence. The emission of light by living organisms, as fireflies. / bios (G. life) / lumen (L. light), genit. luminis / escence.

-esis ... A noun-forming suffix, from the Greek *-esis*, denoting *a process, action.*

cata-phor-esis. The movement of a medicinal substance through a tissue under the influence of an electric field. / kata (G. down) / phoresis (G. a being borne) / esis.

eso- ... A Greek prefix meaning *inward, within, inner.*

eso-trop-ia. A deviation of the eye inward, toward the nose. / eso / tropos (G. a turning) / ia (a Latin noun-forming suffix used in names of disorders).

-esophag- ... esophag- ... Latin combining forms, from *oesophagus* (gullet, esophagus), referring to the *esophagus.*

esophago-cele. A protrusion or herniation of the esophagus. / oesophagus / kele (G. rupture, hernia).

-esthes- ... -esthesi- ... esthesio- ... esthet- ... Greek combining forms, from *aisthesis* (perception), referring to *sensation, feeling, perception.*

an-esthet-ic. Without sensation or feeling. / an (without) / aisthesis / ic (an adjective-forming suffix meaning *marked or characterized by*). *Note:* the combining form *esthet* is more directly related to *aisthetikos* (G. sensitive).

estra-...   estri-...   estro-...   Greek combining forms, from *oistros* (keen desire), referring to the *sexual urge, heat in animals, estrus.*

estro-genic. Producing estrus. / oistros / gen (G. that which produces) / ic (an adjective-forming suffix).

ethn-...   ethno-...   Greek combining forms, from *ethnos* (people, nation), meaning *a basic group of mankind, people.*

ethno-logy. The science that deals with the comparative cultures of peoples. / ethnos / logia (G. study), from logos (word, study).

etic...   A adjective-forming suffix, from the Greek *-etikos*, denoting *a quality, characteristic, feature.*

poly-phyl-etic. Showing the characteristics of several ancestral types. / polys (G. many) / phyle (G. tribe) / etic.

eu-...   A Greek combining form, from *eu* (well), meaning *good, normal, well, easily.*

eu-gen-ics. The science of improving the physical and mental qualities of the human race. / eu / genes (G. born) / ikos (a noun-forming suffix, from the Greek, used to designate a *field of study*).

eury-...   A Greek prefix, from *eurys* (wide), meaning *wide, broad.*

eury-cephal-ic. Having a wide head. / eurys / kephale (G. head) / ic (an adjective-forming suffix meaning *characterized by*).

ex-...   A prefix of Greek origin meaning *out, from, forth, away from, without, thoroughly,* depending on the combining forms with which it is joined.

ex-acerb-ate. To intensify in severity. / ex (here used as an intensifier) / acerbus (L. harsh) / ate (a Latin verb-forming suffix meaning *to become*).

exo- ... A Greek prefix, from *exo* (outside), meaning *outside, outward, external, outer.*

exo-crine. Secreting to the outside or outwardly. / cxo / krinein (G. to separate).

extero- ... A Latin prefix, from *exter* (outside), meaning *outside, external.*

extero-cept-ive. Responding to stimuli from the external environment. / exter / receptus (past participle of *recipere*, receive) / ive (a Latin adjective-forming suffix meaning *having the quality of*).

extra- ... **extro-** ... Latin prefixes, from *extra* (outside of), meaning *outside of, beyond, in addition.*

extra-vas-ation. An outflow of blood from a blood vessel. / extra / vas (L. a vessel) / ation (a Latin noun-forming suffix denoting an *action*).

F

-faci- ... **facio-** ... Latin combining forms, from *facies* (face), referring to the *face, appearance, aspect.*

cranio-faci-al. Pertaining to the cranium and the face. / kranion (G. skull) / facies / al (a Latin adjective-forming suffix).

-facient ... A Latin suffix, from *facere* (to make), present participle *faciens,* genit. *facientis,* meaning *inducing, causing, making.*

somni-facient. A substance inducing sleep. / somnus (L. sleep) / facientis.

-faction ... A Latin suffix, from *facere,* past participle *factus* (to make), meaning *process of making.*

rube-faction. The process of making red, as the skin. / ruber (L. red) / factus / ion (a noun-forming suffix indicating a *process*).

-fasci- ... **fascio-** ... Latin combining forms, from *fascia* (band), referring to *fascia, band or sheet of fibrous tissue.*

extra-fasci-al. Situated outside a fascia. / extra (L. outside) / fascia / al (a Latin objective forming suffix).

febr- ... **febri-** ... **febro-** ... Latin combining forms, from *febris* (fever), meaning *fever, pyrexia.*

febri-fuge. A medicine, or any agent, which reduces fever. / febris / fugere (L. to flee).

-fec-...   feca-...   feci-...   feco-...   Latin combining forms, from *faex*, genit. *faecis* (excrement), referring to *feces, excrement, dung, dregs.*

feca-lith. A concretion or "stone" formed from fecal matter. / faex, faecis / lithos (G. stone).

-femor-...   femori-...   femoro-...   Latin combining forms, from *femur*, genit. *femoris* (thigh), meaning *femur, thighbone.*

retro-femor-al. Situated behind the femur. / retro (L. behind) / femur, femoris / al (a Latin adjective-forming suffix).

-fer-...   -ferous...   -ferr-...   Combining forms, derived from the Latin *ferre* (to bear), meaning to *carry, bring, convey, conduct.*

af-fer-ent. Carrying something toward a particular region or structure. / ferre / ent (a Latin adjective-forming suffix meaning *performing the action of*).

ferr-...   ferri-...   ferro-...   Latin combining forms, from *ferrum* (iron), referring to *iron*. *Note:* "ferri" refers to trivalent iron; "ferro" refers to divalent iron.

ferr-ated. Impregnated with iron. / ferrum / ate (a Latin verb-forming suffix meaning *to treat with*).

fet-...   feti-...   feto-...   Latin combining forms, from *fetus* (offspring), meaning *fetus, newborn.*

feti-cide. The destruction or killing of a fetus. / fetus / caedere (L. cut, kill).

fibrill-...   fibrillo-...   Latin combining forms, from *fibrilla* (small filament), meaning *fibril, minute filament or fiber.*

fibrill-ar. Pertaining to fibrils or fibrillae. / fibrilla / ar (a Latin adjective-forming suffix).

fibr-...   fibra-...   fibri-...   fibro-...   Latin combining forms, from *fibra* (fiber), referring to a *fiber, threadlike structure.*

fibr-oma. A tumor composed of fibrous tissue. / fibra / oma (G. tumor).

-fibrin-...   fibrino-...   Latin combining forms, from *fibra* (fiber), referring to *fibrin.*

fibrino-lysin. An enzyme which aids in the digestion of fibrin. / fibra / lysis (G. a loosening).

fil-...   filar-...   filari-...   Latin combining forms, from *filum* (thread) and *filare* (to spin a thread), meaning *thread, threadworm.*

filar-iasis. Infestation with threadworms. / filare / iasis (a suffix denoting an abnormal condition).

fistul-...   fistula-...   fistuli-...   fistulo-...   Latin combining forms, from *fistula* (a pipe), referring to an *abnormal channel, fistula.*

fistul-ec-tom-y. The surgical excision of a fisulta. / fistula / ek (G. out) / temnein (G. cut) / y (a suffix indicating an action).

flagell-...   flagelli-...   flagello-...   Latin combining form from *flagellum* (whip), referring to a *whiplike process, flagellum.*

flagelli-form. Shaped like a flagellum or whip. / flagellum / forma (L. shape, form).

flatul-...   flatulo-...   Latin combining forms, based on *flare* (to blow), past participle *flatus,* and *flatulentus* (flatulence), referring to the presence of *gas in the intestinal tract, distention caused by gas.*

flatulo-lyt-ic. / flatulentus / lytos (G. dissolvable) / ic (an adjective-forming suffix).

flav-... flavi-... flavo-... Latin combining forms, from *flavus* (yellow), meaning *yellow.*

flav-escent. Turning yellow. / flavus / escent (an adjective-forming suffix meaning *becoming, turning into*).

-flect-... -flex-... Combining forms, derived from the Latin *flectere* (to bend) and *flexus* (bent), meaning to *curve, flex, bend.*

genu-flect. To bend the knee, as in worship. / genu (L. knee) / flectere (bend).

retro-flex-ion. A bending backward of an organ, as the uterus. / retro (L. backward) / flexus / ion (a suffix forming nouns).

follicul-... A Latin combining form, from *folliculus* (small sac), meaning *a follicle, small bag, gland.*

follicul-itis. Inflammation of follicles. / folliculus / itis (a Greek suffix denoting *inflammation*).

-form... A Latin combining form, from *forma* (form), meaning *form, shape, image.*

digiti-form. Shaped like a finger. / digitus (L. finger, toe) / forma.

fragil-... fragili-... fragilo-... Latin combining forms, from *fragilis* (easily broken), meaning *brittle, fragile.*

fragilo-cyte. A red blood cell which is abnormally fragile. / fragilis / kytos (G. cell).

fract-... fracto-... fracturo-... Combining forms, derived from the Latin *frangere* (to break), past participle *fractus* (broken), denoting a reference to a *fracture* or *break.*

dif-fract-ion. The breaking up of a ray of light into its constituent parts. / dis (L. away) / fractus (broken) / ion (a suffix forming nouns). *Note:* the *s* of the prefix *dis* is changed into an *f* when the following letter is an *f*.

fracturo-graphy. The taking of x-ray pictures of a fractured bone. / fractus / graphein (G. to write, record).

front- ...   **fronti-** ...   **fronto-** ...   Latin combining forms, from *frons,* genit. *frontis* (forehead), meaning *front, anterior, forehead.*

fronti-petal. Moving to the front. / frons, frontis / petere (L. to seek).

fruct- ...   **fructi-** ...   **fructo-** ...   Latin combining forms, from *fructus* (fruit, enjoyment), referring to *fruit, fructose.*

fructi-fer-ous. Bearing or producing fruit. / fructus / ferre (L. to bear) / ous (a Latin adjective-forming suffix).

frugi- ...   A Latin combining form, from *frux,* genit. *frugis* (fruit), meaning *fruit.*

frugi-vor-ous. Eating mainly fruit. / frux, frugis / vorare (L. to devour) / ous (a Latin adjective-forming suffix).

-fug- ...   **-fugal** ...   **-fuge** ...   Combining forms, derived from the Latin *fugere* (to flee), denoting a reference to *driving away, moving away, fleeing.*

vermi-fuge. A medicinal substance, or any agent, which expels intestinal worms. / vermis (L. worm) / fuge (a Latin suffix indicating something that *drives away* or *out*).

-funct- ...   **function-** ...   Latin combining forms, from *fungi* (to perform), *functio* (performance), referring to *function, performance.*

hypo-function. Decreased function. / hypo (G. less than) / functio.

fund- ...   **fundi-** ...   **fundo-** ...   **fundu-** ...   Combining forms, derived from the Latin *fundus* (bottom), referring to a *base* or *bottom,* as of an organ.

fund-ectom-y. The surgical excision of the base of an organ. / fund (base) / ektome (G. cut out) / y (a noun-forming suffix).

fundu-scope. An instrument used for examining the fundus or base of the eyeball. / fundu / skopein (G. examine).

fung-... fungi-... fungo-... Latin combining forms, from *fungus* (mushroom), meaning *fungus.*

fungi-cide. A substance capable of destroying fungi. / fungus / cide, caedere (G. to kill).

-fy... A verb-forming suffix, from the Latin *facere* (to make), meaning *to make, cause to be or become.*

lique-fy. To cause to become a liquid. / liquere (L. to be liquid) / fy.

G

-galact-...   galacta-...   galacto-...   Greek combining forms, from *gala,* genit. *galaktos* (milk), meaning *milk.*

galacto-phag-ous. Subsisting on milk. / galaktos / phagein (G. to eat) / ous (an adjective-forming suffix).

galvan-...   galvani-...   galvano-...   Eponymic combining forms, based on Luigi *Galvani,* Italian physicist, referring to *direct current, galvanic electricity.*

galvano-cautery. Cautery by means of direct current. / Galvani / kaiein (G. to burn).

gam-...   gamo-...   -gamy...   Greek combining forms, from *gamos* (marriage), meaning *marriage, sexual union.*

endo-gam-y. Marriage within one's tribe. / endon (G. within) / gamos / y (a noun-forming suffix indicating a *condition*).

gamet-...   gameto-...   Greek combining forms, from *gamete* (wife), referring to a *reproductive cell, gamete, malarial parasite.*

gameto-cyte. A cell capable of producing gametes. / gamete / kytos (G. cell).

gangli-...   ganglio-...   ganglion-...   gangliono-...   Greek combining forms, from *ganglion* (knot), referring to a *ganglion, group of nerve cells.*

ganglion-ated. Having a ganglion or ganglia. / ganglion / ated (a suffix meaning *provided with, characterized by*).

gastr- ... **gastri-** ... **gastro-** ... Greek combining forms, from *gaster* (stomach), genit. *gastros,* meaning *stomach.*

gastro-enter-itis. Inflammation of the stomach and the intestine. / gaster / enteron (G. intestine) / itis (a suffix used to denote *inflammation*).

gelatin- ... **gelatini-** ... **gelatino-** ... Latin combining forms, from *gelare,* past participle *gelata* (congeal, freeze), referring to *gelatin, gel, jelly.*

gelatino-lyt-ic. Capable of dissolving gelatin. / gelata / lytos (dissolvable) / ic (an adjective-forming suffix).

gemell- ... **gemelli-** ... **gemello-** ... Latin combining forms, from *gemellus,* diminutive of *geminus* (twin), meaning *twin, twins, twinning.*

gemello-logy. The study of twinning. / gemellus / logia (a study, from the Greek *logos,* word, study).

-gemin- ... **gemini-** ... **gemino-** ... Latin combining forms, from *geminus* (twin), meaning *twin, twins, twinning.*

bi-gemin-al. Paired; consisting of two; double. / bis (L. twice) / geminus / al (an adjective-forming suffix meaning *having the characteristics of*).

-gen ... A Latin terminal combining form, from *generare* (beget, produce), used to form nouns which denote a *producer, something that produces.*

pyro-gen. Something producing fever. / pyr, genit. pyros (G. fire, heat) / generare.

-gener- ... A Latin combining form, from *generare* (beget), meaning *beget, produce, originate, cause.*

con-gener-ous. Allied in origin. / con, com (a prefix meaning *to-gether*) / generare / ous (a Latin suffix meaning *characterized by*).

geni-... genio-... geny-... genyo-... Combining forms, derived from the Greek *geneion* (chin) and genys (lower jaw), referring to the *chin* or *lower jaw*.

micro-gen-ia. Abnormal smallness of the chin. / mikros (G. small) / geneion (chin) / ia (a Latin noun-forming suffix denoting a *condition*).

genit-... genito-... Latin combining forms, from *genitus,* past participle of *gignere* (to beget), referring to *reproduction, sexual organs, birth.*

genit-al-ia. The sexual or reproductive organs. / genitus / al (an adjective-forming suffix) / ia (a noun-forming suffix used, in some cases, to form plurals).

geno-... A Greek combining form, from *genos* (race), referring to *race, kind, sex.*

geno-type. A typical species of a genus. / genos / typos (G. model, figure).

genu-... A Latin combining form, from *genu* (knee), meaning *knee.*

genu-cubit-al. Pertaining to the knees and the elbows. / genu / cubitum (L. elbow) / al (a Latin adjective-forming suffix).

geo-... A combining form, derived from the Greek *ge* (earth), referring to the *earth, soil, dirt.*

geo-phag-ia. The eating of earth or turf. / ge (earth) / phagein (G. to eat) / ia (a Latin noun-forming suffix used in names of disorders).

ger-... gerat-... geri-... gerio-... gero-... geronto-... Greek combining forms, from *geras* (old age) and *geron,* genit. *gerontos* (old man), referring to *old age, elderly person.*

ger-iatric. Pertaining to the treatment of the elderly. / geron / iatros (G. physician) / ic (an adjective-forming suffix meaning *pertaining to*).

germin- ...   **germino-** ...   **germo-** ...   Latin combining forms, from *germen* (offshoot), meaning *sprout, bud, embryo, primordium.*

germin-ation. The beginning of growth; a sprouting. / germen / ation (a noun-forming suffix denoting a *process*).

-geus- ...   **-geusia** ...   Greek combining forms, from *geusis* (taste), referring to *taste, sense of taste.*

hypo-geus-ia. Dullness of the sense of taste. / hypo (a Greek prefix meaning *less than*) / geusis / ia (a noun-forming suffix used in names of disorders).

giga- ...   **gigant-** ...   **giganto-** ...   Greek combining forms, from *gigas*, genit. *gigantos* (giant), meaning *gigantic, huge, a billion.*

giganto-cyte. A very large red blood cell. / gigantos / kytos (G. cell).

gingiv- ...   **gingivo-** ...   Latin combining forms, from *gingiva* (gum), meaning *gum.*

gingiv-ec-tom-y. Surgical excision of a portion of the gum. / gingiva / ek (G. out) / temnein (G. to cut) / y (a noun-forming suffix indicating a *process*).

gland- ...   **glandi-** ...   Latin combining forms, from *glans*, genit. *glandis* (acorn), meaning *gland.*

glandi-lemma. A membrane surrounding a gland. / glans, glandis / lemma (G. husk, covering).

gli- ...   **-glia** ...   **glio-** ...   Greek combining forms, from *glia* (glue), referring to a *glue-like tissue, neuroglia.*

gli-osis. Abnormal growth of neuroglia. / glia / osis (a Greek noun-forming suffix denoting an *abnormal condition*).

glob-...   **globul-**...   **globuli-**...   **globulo-**...   Combining forms, derived from the Latin *globus* (ball) and *globulus* (small ball), referring to a *sphere, globe, drop, ball.*

glob-ose. Having a spherical form. / glob (sphere) / ose (a suffix meaning *resembling*).

globulo-lytic. Destructive to red blood cells. / globulo (an allusion to the roundness of red blood cells) / lysis (G. a loosening), lytikos (loosing).

glom-...   **glomerul-**...   **glomerulo-**...   Latin combining forms, from *glomus*, diminutive *glomerulus* (ball), referring to the *glomerulus of the kidney.*

glomerulo-nephr-itis. Inflammation of the kidney and the glomeruli. / glomerulus / nephros (G. kidney) / itis (a suffix indicating *inflammation*).

gloss-...   **glosso-**...   Greek combining forms, from *glossa* (tongue), meaning *tongue, tonguelike structure.*

glosso-pleg-ia. Paralysis of the tongue. / glossa / plege (G. stroke) / ia (a noun-forming suffix denoting a *disorder*).

glott-...   **glotto-**...   Greek combining forms, from the Attic Greek *glotta* (tongue), meaning *tongue, tonguelike structure.*

glotto-logy. The medical science of the tongue. / glotta / logy (G. *logia*, a science).

gluc-...   **gluco-**...   Greek combining forms, from *glykys* (sweet), referring to *glucose, sugar, sweetness.*

gluco-genesis. The formation of glucose. / glykys / genesis (G. origin).

glyc-...   **glyco-**...   **glycogen-**...   Greek combining forms, from *glykys* (sweet), meaning *sugar, carbohydrate, glycogen.*

hyper-glyc-em-ia. An increase in blood sugar. / hyper (in excess) / glykys / haima (G. blood) / ia (a noun-forming suffix used in names of *disorders*).

glycer-...   glycerin-...   glycero-... Greek combining forms, from *glykeros* (sweet), referring to *glycerin, glycerol.*

glycero-phil-ic. Combining readily with glycerin. / glykeros / philein (G. to love) / ic (an adjective-forming suffix).

-glyph-...   glypho-... Greek combining forms, from *glyphein* (to carve), referring to *carving, a carving.*

hiero-glyph-ic. An ancient writing in which a picture represents a word, syllable, or sound. / hieros (G. sacred) / glyph / ic (a noun-forming suffix).

glypt-...   glypto-... Greek combining forms, from *glyptos* (carved), meaning *carved.*

glypto-graphy. The study of carved stones. / glyptos / graphia (G. writing, from *graphein*, to write).

gnath-...   gnatho-... Greek combining forms, from *gnathos* (jaw), referring to the *jaw, jawbone.*

a-gnath-ia. The condition of having no lower jaw. / a (without) / gnathos / ia (a Latin noun-forming suffix used in names of *disorders*).

-gnomy... A terminal combining form, from the Greek *gnome* (judgment, intelligence), referring to the ability to *judge, determine.*

physio-gnomy. The judgment of mental quality by observing facial features. / physis (G. nature) / gnomy.

-gnosia...   -gnosis...   -gnostic... Greek combining forms, from *gnosis* (knowledge), meaning *knowledge, recognition, appreciation.*

baro-gnosis. The ability to perceive or recognize weight. / baros (G. weight) / gnosis.

-gon-...   gone-...   gono-... Greek combining forms, from *gone* (a seed), referring to *semen, sperm, seed.*

gono-cyte. An early or primitive reproductive cell. / gone / kytos (G. cell).

gon- . . .   **gone-** . . .   **gony-** . . .   Greek combining forms, from *gony* (knee), meaning *knee.*

gony-campsis. An abnormal bending of the knee. / gony / kampsis (G. a bending).

gonad- . . .   **gonado-** . . .   Latin combining forms, from *gonas* (organ of reproductive cells), plural *gonades,* referring to a *testicle, ovary, gonad.*

gonado-therap-y. Treatment with hormones from the ovary or testis. / gonades / therapeuein (G. to treat) / y (a noun-forming suffix denoting an *action*).

gonecyst- . . .   **gonecysto-** . . .   Greek combining forms, from *gone* (seed) and *kystis* (sac, bladder), meaning *seminal vesicle.*

gone-cyst-alg-ia. / gone / kystis / algos (G. pain) / ia (a noun-forming suffix used in names of *diseases*)

goni- . . .   **gonio-** . . .   Combining forms, derived from the Greek *gonia* (angle), referring to an *angle, corner.*

gonio-meter. An instrument used to measure angles. / gonio (angle) / metron (G. to measure).

goni-al. Pertaining to an angle. / goni (angle) / al (an adjective-forming suffix meaning *pertaining to.*

grad- . . .   **gradi-** . . .   **-grade** . . .   Latin combining forms, from *gradi* (to walk), meaning *walk, step.*

planti-grade. Walking on the entire sole of the foot. / planta (L. sole of the foot) / gradi.

-gram . . .   A Greek suffix, from *gramma* (something written), denoting a *tracing, recording, writing, letter.*

encephalo-gram. An x-ray picture of the brain. / en (in) / kephale (G. head) / gram.

granul-... **granuli-**... **granulo-**... Latin combining forms, from *granulum* (small grain), referring to a *granule, small particle*.

granulo-cyte. A blood cell containing granules. / granulum / kytos (G. cell).

-graph-... **grapho-**... **-graphy**... Greek combining forms, from *graphein* (to write), referring to *writing, recording, recorder*.

a-graph-ia. Loss of the normal ability to write. / a (negative, no) / graphein / ia (a noun-forming suffix used in names of *disorders*).

electro-cardio-graph. An instrument for recording the electric current produced by the contraction of the heart. / electro (a combining form referring to electricity, from the Greek *elektron,* amber) / kardia (G. heart) / graph (a terminal combining form meaning *that which writes or records, from graphein*).

-gravid-... **-gravida**... **gravido-**... Latin combining forms, from *gravida* (heavy), meaning *pregnant, pregnancy*.

multi-gravida. A pregnant woman who has been pregnant two or more times before. / multus (L. many) / gravida (pregnant; heavy with child).

-gust-... **gustat-**... Latin combining forms, from *gustare* (to taste), past participle *gustatus*, referring to *taste, sense of taste*.

gustat-ory. Pertaining to, or involving, the sense of taste. / gustatus / ory (a Latin suffix meaning *pertaining to*).

gymno-... Greek combining form, from *gymnos* (naked), meaning *naked, uncovered, exposed*.

gymno-scopo-phil-ia. A compelling desire to look at naked bodies, usually of the opposite sex. / gymnos / skopein (G. to see) / philein (G. to love) / ia (a noun-forming suffix).

gyn- ...   **gyne-** ...   **gyneco-** ...   **gyno-** ...   Greek combining forms, from *gyne* and *gynaikos* (woman), meaning *woman, female.*

gyne-phob-ia. Fear of, or aversion for, women. / gyne / phobos (G. fear) / ia (a noun-forming suffix denoting a *disorder*).

gyneco-mast-ia. Excessive development of the breast in a male. / gynaikos / mastos (G. breast) / ia (a noun-forming suffix denoting an *abnormality*).

-gyr- ...   **gyro-** ...   Combining forms, derived from the Greek *gyros* (a circle) or from the Latin *gyrare*, present participle *gyratus* (to turn), denoting a reference to a *circle, rotation, ring.*

oculo-gyr-ic. Pertaining to, or involving, rotation of the eyeball. / oculus (L. eye) / gyrare (L. turn) / ic (a Latin adjective-forming suffix).

H

hagi-... **hagio-**... Greek combining forms, from *hagios* (holy), meaning *sacred, holy, saintly.*

hagio-therapy. Healing by a holy man. / hagios / therapeia (G. therapy).

-hal-... **halit-**... Combining forms, derived from the Latin *halare* (to breathe) and *halitus* (breath), referring to the *process of breathing* and *breath.*

ex-hal-ation. The process of breathing out. / ex (L. out) / halare (breathe) / ation (a noun-forming suffix denoting a *process* or *action*).

halit-osis. Unpleasant breath. / halitus (breath) / osis (a Greek suffix denoting a *condition,* usually abnormal).

halluc-... **halluci-**... **halluco-**... Latin combining forms, from *hallux* (great toe), genit. *hallucis,* referring to the *great toe.*

halluci-form. Resembling the great toe. / hallucis / forma (L. form, shape).

halo-... A Greek combining form, from *hals* (G. salt), genit. *halos,* referring to the *sea, salt, halogens.*

halo-biont. An organism thriving in salt water. / halos / biont (a Greek noun-forming suffix denoting *an organism having a specified mode of life*).

hapl-... **haplo-**... Greek combining forms, from *haploos* (simple, single), meaning *simple, single.*

haplo-dermat-itis. Simple or uncomplicated dermatitis. / haploos / derma (G. skin), genit. *dermatos* / itis (a suffix denoting inflammation).

hapt-... **hapto-**... Greek combining forms, from *haptein* (to touch), meaning *touch, seizure, contact.*

hapto-met-er. An instrument used to test sensitivity to touch. / haptein / metron (G. measure) / er (a suffix denoting a thing performing a given *function*).

hecto-... A Greek combining form, from *hekaton* (hundred), meaning *one hundred.*

hecto-gram. A weight equal to 100 grams. / hekaton / gramma (G. small weight).

hel-... **hela-**... **helo-**... Combining forms, derived from the Greek *helos* (head of nail), referring to a *callus, corn.*

hel-osis. The presence of corns or calluses. / helos (corn, callus) / osis (a Greek noun-forming suffix denoting an *abnormal condition*).

helc-... **helco-**... Greek combining forms, from *helkos* (ulcer), meaning *ulcer, ulceration.*

helc-ec-tom-y. The surgical excision of an ulcer. / helkos / ek (out) / tome (G. a cutting) / y (a noun-forming suffix denoting an *action*).

heli-... **helio-**... Greek combining forms, from *helios* (sun), referring to *sunlight, sun.*

helio-trop-ism. Tropism caused by sunlight; a turning toward the sun. / helios / tropos (G. a turning) / ism (a noun-forming suffix denoting an *act*).

helminth-...   helminthi-...   helmintho-...   Greek combining forms, from *helmins* (a worm), genit. *helminthos,* referring to a *parasitic worm.*

helminth-iasis. Infestation with parasitic worms. / helminthos / iasis (a suffix denoting a diseased condition or infestation).

hemi-...   A Greek prefix, from *hemi* (half), meaning *half.*

hemi-faci-al. Affecting half or one side of the face. / hemi / facies (L. face) / al (an adjective-forming suffix).

hemoglobin-...   hemoglobini-...   hemoglobino-...   Combining forms derived from the Greek *haima* (blood) and the Latin *globin* (a protein), referring to *hemoglobin, the red pigment of blood.*

hemoglobin-em-ia. The presence of hemoglobin in blood plasma. / haima / globin / haima / ia (a Latin noun-forming suffix used in names of *diseases*).

hemorrhoid-...   hemorrhoidi-...   hemorrhoido-...   Greek combining forms, from *haima* (blood) and *rhein* (flow), referring to *hemorrhoids. Note:* The Greek term for hemorrhoids was *haimorrhoides phlebes,* bleeding veins.

hemorrhoid-ek-tom-y. / haima / rhein / ek (G. out) / temnein (G. cut) / y (a suffix denoting an *action*).

hepat-...   hepatico-...   hepato-...   Greek combining forms, from *hepar,* genit. *hepatos* (liver), meaning *liver.*

hepato-lith. A calculus or "stone" found in the liver. / hepar, hepatos / lithos (G. stone).

hept-...   hepta-...   Greek combining forms, from *hepta* (seven), meaning *seven.*

hepta-dactyl-ia. The condition of having seven digits on one limb. / hepta / daktylos (G. finger) / ia (a noun-forming suffix used in names of *disorders*).

heredit- . . .   A Latin combining form, from *hereditas* (heirship), meaning *heredity*.

heredit-ary. Pertaining to, or involving, inheritance. / hereditas / ary (an adjective-forming suffix meaning *pertaining to*).

heredo- . . .   A Latin combining form, from *heres* (heir), genit. *heredis*, meaning *hereditary*.

heredo-path-ia. An inherited disease. / heres, heredis / pathos (disease) / ia (a Latin noun-forming suffix used in names of *diseases*).

hermaphrodit- . . .   A Greek combining form, from *Hermes* (Greek god) and *Aphrodite* (Greek goddess of love), referring to *hermaphroditism*.

hermaphrodit-ic. Of the nature of a hermaphrodite. / Hermes / Aphrodite / ic (a Latin adjective-forming suffix).

herni- . . .   **hernio-** . . .   Latin combining forms, from *hernia* (rupture), referring to a *hernia*.

herni-clit-ic. Inclined to be affected with a hernia. / hernia / klinein (G. incline) / ic (a Latin adjective-forming suffix).

herpes- . . .   **herpet-** . . .   **herpeti-** . . .   **herpeto-** . . .   Greek combining forms, from *herpein*, genit. *herpetis* (to creep), meaning *herpes*.

herpeti-form. Resembling herpes. / herpetis / forma (L. form, shape).

heter- . . .   **hetero-** . . .   Greek combining forms, from *heteros* (other), meaning *other, another, different*.

heter-esthes-ia. The condition of having different sensations in adjoining regions of the skin. / heteros / aisthesis (G. perception) / ia (a noun-forming suffix denoting a *condition*).

hex- . . .   **hexa-** . . .   Greek combining forms, from *hex* (six), meaning *six, sixfold*.

hex-ose. A sugar containing six carbon atoms. / hex / ose (a suffix denoting a sugar, from the Greek gleuk*os*, sweet).

-hex- ... **-hexi-** ... **-hexis** ... Combining forms, derived from the Greek *hexis* (habit, condition), referring to *condition, habit.*

cac-hex-ia. A condition of ill health. / kakos (G. bad) / hexis (condition) / ia (a suffix used to form nouns indicating *diseases, conditions*).

-hidr- ... **hidro-** ... **hidrot-** ... Greek combining forms, from *hidros* (sweat) and *hidrotikos* (causing sweating), referring to *sweat, sweating, perspiration.*

an-hidrot-ic. A substance which checks perspiration. / an (without) / hidrotikos / ic (an adjective-forming suffix denoting a *property*).

hier- ... **hiero-** ... Greek combining forms, from *hieros* (holy, sacred), meaning *holy, sacred, religious, religion.*

hiero-therapy. Treatment of disease by religious rites. / hieros / therapeia (G. therapy).

hippo- ... A Greek combining form, from *hippos* (horse), meaning *horse.*

hippo-campus. A ridge along the lateral ventricle of the brain. / hippos / kampos (G. sea monster).

hist- ... **histi-** ... **histio-** ... **histo-** ... Greek combining forms, from *histos* (web), meaning *web, tissue.*

hist-affine. Having an affinity for tissues. / histos / affinis (L. adjacent).

hodo- ... A Greek combining form, from *hodos* (way, road), denoting a *road, path, way.*

hodo-phobia. Abnormal fear of travel. / hodos / phobos (G. fear) / ia (a noun-forming suffix denoting an abnormal *condition*).

hod-. . .   hodo-. . .   Greek combining forms, from *hodos* (path), meaning *pathway, nerve path.*

hodo-neuro-mere. A segment of the trunk with its nerves (in embryology). / hodos / neuron (G. nerve) / meros (G. part).

hol-. . .   holo-. . .   Greek combining forms, from *holos* (entire), meaning *whole, entire, exclusively.*

holo-gyn-ic. Transmitted exclusively through the female line, as certain diseases. / holos (entire) / gyne (G. woman) / ic (an adjective-forming suffix).

homal-. . .   homali-. . .   homalo-. . .   Greek combining forms, from *homalos* (even), meaning *level, even, smooth.*

homalo-cephal-us. A person having a flat head. / homalos / kephale (G. head) / us (a noun-forming suffix meaning *one who*). . .

homeo-. . .   homo-. . .   homoio-. . .   Greek combining forms, from *homoios* (like) and *homos* (same), referring to *sameness, similarity, unchanging condition.*

homeo-morph-ous. Similar or like in form. / homoios / morphe (G. form) / ous (an adjective-forming suffix meaning *having*).

horm-. . .   hormon-. . .   hormono-. . .   Greek combining forms, from *hormaein* (excite), meaning *spur, urge, set in motion, excite, hormone.*

hormon-agogue. A substance which stimulates the secretion of a hormone. / hormaein / agogos (G. leader).

humer-. . .   humero-. . .   Latin combining forms, from *humerus* (shoulder), referring to the *humerus, bone of upper arm.*

scapulo-humer-al. Pertaining to the shoulder blade and the humerus. / scapula (L. shoulder blade) / humerus / al (a Latin adjective-forming suffix).

hyal-. . .   hyalo-. . .   Greek combining forms, from *hyalos* (glass), meaning *glass, glassy, translucent.*

hyal-oid. Resembling glass. / hyalos / oeides (G. resembling).

hydatid-...   **hydatidi-**...   **hydatido-**...   Greek combining forms, from *hydatis,* genit. *hydatidos* (a watery vesicle), referring to a *hydatid cyst* or *hydatids.*

hydatidi-form. Having the form of a hydatid cyst. / hydatis, hydatidos / forma (L. form).

-hydr-...   **hydro-**...   Greek combining forms, from *hydor* (water), referring to *water, fluid, hydrogen.*

hydr-arthr-osis. The presence of fluid in a joint. / hydor / arthron (G. joint) / osis (a noun-forming suffix denoting a *disorder*).

hydrargyr-...   **hydrargyro-**...   Greek combining forms, from *hydor* (water, liquid) and *argyros* (silver), meaning *mercury.*

hydr-argyro-mania. A mental disorder caused by mercury poisoning. / hydor / argyros / mania (G. madness).

hyet-...   **hyeto-**...   Greek combining forms, from *hyetos* (rain), meaning *rain, rainfall.*

hyeto-metr-y. The measurement of rainfall. / hyetos / metron (G. measure) / y (a noun-forming suffix denoting an *action*).

hygien-...   **hygio-**...   Greek combining forms, from *hygieinos* (healthful), referring to *health, hygiene.*

hygien-ist. A practitioner of hygiene. / hygieinos / ist (a noun-forming suffix denoting a specified *practitioner*).

hygr-...   **hygro-**...   Greek combining forms, from *hygros* (wet), referring to *moisture, humidity, dampness, fluid.*

hygr-oma. A tumor formed by an accumulation of fluid. / hygros / oma (G. tumor).

hyl-...   **hyle-**...   **hylo-**...   Greek combining forms, from *hyle* (matter), meaning *matter, substance, material.*

bio-hylo-trop-ic. Affecting living matter. / bios (G. life) / hyle / trope (G. a turn) / ic (an adjective-forming suffix).

hymen-...   hymeno-...   Greek combining forms, from *hymen* (membrane), meaning *hymen, membrane.*

hymeno-tom-y. A surgical cutting of the hymen. / hymen / tome (G. a cutting) / y (a noun-forming suffix denoting an action).

hyo-...   hyoid-...   Greek combining forms, from *hyoeides* (like the letter upsilon), referring to the *hyoid bone.*

hyo-gloss-al. Pertaining to the hyoid bone and the tongue. / hyoeides / glossa (G. tongue) / al (an adjective-forming suffix).

hyper-...   A Greek prefix, from *hyper* (above), having several meanings, especially *above, excessive, more than normal, over.*

hyper-calc-em-ia. The presence of an excess of calcium in the blood. / hyper (above) / calx (L. lime) / haima (G. blood) / ia (a noun-forming suffix used in names of *disorders*).

-hypn-...   hypno-...   Greek combining forms, from *hypnos* (sleep), referring to *sleep, hypnotism.*

hypno-ana-lysis. Psychoanalysis performed while the patient is hypnotized. / hypnos / ana (G. throughout) / lysis (G. a loosing).

hypo-...   A prefix, derived from the Greek *hypo* (under), meaning *less than normal, under, below, beneath.*

hypo-derm-ic. Administered beneath the skin, as an injection. / hypo (beneath) / derma (G. skin) / ic (an adjective-forming suffix).

hypo-therm-ia. An abnormally low body temperature. / hypo / therme (G. heat) / ia (a noun-forming suffix).

hyps-...   hypso-...   Greek combining forms, from *hypsos* (height), referring to *elevation, height.*

hypso-phob-ia. Fear of high places. / hypsos / phobos (G. fear) / ia (a Latin noun-forming suffix used in names of *disorders*).

hyster-...   **hysteri-**...   **hystero-**...   Greek combining forms, from *hystera* (uterus), referring to the *uterus*.

hyster-ec-tom-y. Excision of the uterus. / hystera / ek (out) / tome (G. a cutting) / y (a noun-forming suffix denoting an *action*).

I

-ia . . .   A noun-forming suffix, from the Latin *-ia,* used to denote *names of disorders, diseases, biological classes.*

hemat-ur-ia. The presence of blood in the urine. / haima, genit. haimatos (G. blood) / ouron (G. urine) / ia.

-iasis . . .   A terminal combining form, from the Latin or Greek, denoting a *process* or *condition,* especially a *pathological condition.*

mydr-iasis. An abnormal dilatation of the pupil. / mydros (G. a mass of red-hot metal) / iasis.

iatr- . . .   **iatro-** . . .   Greek combining forms, from *iatros* (physician), referring to *physicians, medicine, treatment.*

iatro-genic. Caused by a physician. / iatros / gen (a Greek suffix, from *gignesthai,* to be born, meaning *that which produces*) / ic (an adjective-forming suffix meaning *pertaining to*).

-ible . . .   An adjective-forming suffix, from the Latin *-ibilis,* meaning *able to, capable of being.*

re-frang-ible. That may be refracted, as light rays. / re (back) / frangere (L. to break) / ible.

-ic . . .   1. An adjective-forming suffix, from the Latin *-icus,* meaning *pertaining to, resembling, of the nature of, in the manner of, containing, connected with.* 2. A noun-forming suffix denoting *a person or thing having certain characteristics, belonging to, producing, derived from.*

cephal-ic. Pertaining to the head. / kephale (G. head) / ic.

stomach-ic. A medicinal substance which aids digestion. / stomachus (L. stomach) / ic.

-ical . . .   An adjective-forming suffix, from the Latin *-icalis,* denoting *a quality, characteristic.*

patho-log-ical. Involving a disease. / pathos (G. suffering, disease) / logos (G. study) / ical.

Ichthy- . . .   **ichthyo-** . . .   Greek combining forms, from *ichthys* (a fish), meaning *fish, fishlike.*

ichthy-osis. A disease marked by scaliness of the skin. / ichthys / osis (a Greek suffix used in names of *diseases*).

-icity . . .   A noun-forming suffix, from the Latin *-icitas,* denoting *a quality, condition, fact.*

chron-icity. The condition of being chronic. / chronos (G. time) / icity.

icter- . . .   **ictero-** . . .   Greek combining forms, from *ikteros* (jaundice), meaning *jaundice, icterus.*

icter-itious. Affected or marked by jaundice. / ikteros / itious (an adjective-forming suffix meaning characterized by).

-id . . .   An adjective-forming suffix, from the Latin *-idus,* denoting *a quality, characteristic.*

rab-id. Affected with rabies. / rabere (L. to be mad) / id.

ide- . . .   **idea-** . . .   **ideo-** . . .   Greek combining forms, from *idea* (appearance), meaning *idea, concept, impression.*

ide-ation. The formation of ideas. / idea / ation (a Latin suffix used to form nouns denoting an *action, process*).

idio- ...   A Greek prefix, from *idios* (one's own), meaning *personal, alone, distinct, one's own, its own, peculiar to an individual.*

idio-ventricul-ar. Pertaining to, or involving, the ventricles alone. / idios / ventriculus (L. ventricle) / ar (an adjective-forming suffix meaning *pertaining to*).

ign- ...   **igni-** ...   A Latin combining form, from *ignis* (fire), meaning *fire, flame.*

ign-escent. Catching fire easily; bursting into flame. / ignis / escent (an adjective-forming suffix meaning *beginning to be*).

il- ...   A Latin prefix, having the same function as in- *(no, not without)*, used before a word or combining form beginning with the letter *l.*

il-legitim-ate. Not legitimate. / il / legitimus (L. lawful) / ate (a Latin adjective-forming suffix meaning *characterized by*).

-ile ...   1. A noun-forming suffix, from the Latin *-ilis*, denoting *a person or thing having a specified characteristic.* 2. An adjective-forming suffix denoting *suitability, quality, relationship.*

juven-ile. A young person. / juvenis (L. young person) / ile.

vir-ile. Having the vigor of manhood. / vir (L. man) / ile.

ile- ...   **ileo-** ...   Latin combining forms, from *ileum* (ileum), referring to the *ileum, third part of small intestine.*

ileo-cec-al. Pertaining to the ileum and cecum. / ileum / caecus (L. blind) / al (a Latin adjective-forming suffix).

ili- ...   **ilio-** ...   Latin combining forms, from *ilium* (ilium), referring to the *ilium, flank.*

ilio-cost-al. Pertaining to the ilium and the ribs. / ilium / costa (L. rib) / al (an adjective-forming suffix).

-ility ...   A noun-forming suffix, from the Latin *-ilitas*, denoting *a condition, state.*

im-bec-ility. The condition of being an imbecile. / im (without) / baculus (L. a staff used for support) / ility.

im- ...   A Latin prefix, having the same function as in- *(no, not, without)*, used before words or combining forms beginning with the letters *b, m,* or *p.*

im-perforate. Not perforated. / im / perforatus (L. pierced with holes).

immun- ...   **immuni-** ...   **immuno-** ...   Latin combining forms, from *immunis* (exempt), meaning *immunity, security from, resistance against.*

immun-ization. The process of becoming or making immune. / immunis / ization (a Latin noun-forming suffix denoting a *process*).

in- ...   A Latin prefix meaning *in, on, toward, within.*

in-suf-flate. To blow (something) into a body cavity. / in / suf (up from under) / flare, flatus (L. to blow).

in- ...   A Latin prefix meaning *no, not, without.*

in-anim-ate. Not alive. / in / *animare,* past participle *animatus* (L. to make alive) / ate (a Latin adjective-forming suffix meaning *characterized by*).

incis- ...   **inciso-** ...   Latin combining forms, from *incidere,* past participle *incisus* (to cut), meaning *incision, cut, depression, notch.*

in-cis-ion. A cut; the act of cutting. / in (in) / incisus (cut) / ion (a noun-forming suffix indicating an *act*).

incud- ...   **incudi-** ...   **incudo-** ...   Latin combining forms, from *incus,* genit. *incudis* (anvil), referring to the *incus,* one of the ossicles.

incudi-form. Shaped like an anvil; shaped like the incus. / incus, incudis / forma (L. form, shape).

infan-...   infant-...   infanti-...   infanto-...   Latin combining forms, from *infans*, genit. *infantis* (infant), meaning *infant, young child*.

infanti-cide. The killing or murder of an infant. / infans, infantis / caedere (L. to kill).

infra-...   A prefix, derived from the Latin *infra* (beneath), meaning *below, beneath, underneath*.

infra-patell-ar. Situated below the kneecap. / infra (below) / patella (L. a small dish, hence, because of the resemblance, the patella or kneecap) / ar (an adjective-forming suffix meaning *pertaining to*).

infra-clavicular. Situated below the clavicle or collarbone. / infra / clavicula (L. little key, hence, because of the resemblance, the clavicle) / ar.

infundibul-...   infundibuli-...   infundibulo-...   Latin combining forms, from *infundibulum* (funnel), referring to an *infundibulum, funnel-shaped structure*.

infundibuli-form. Shaped like a funnel. / infundibulum / forma (L. shape).

inguin-...   inguino-...   Latin combining forms, from *inguen*, genit. *inguinis* (groin), meaning *groin*.

inguin-al. Pertaining to, or situated in, the groin. / inguinis / al (a Latin adjective-forming suffix meaning *pertaining to*).

inos-...   A Greek combining form, from *is*, genit. *inos* (fiber), referring to *fibrin*.

inos-uria. An increase in the amount of fibrin in the urine. / is, inos / ouron (G. urine) / ia (a noun-forming suffix denoting a *condition*).

insect-...   insecti-...   insecto-...   Latin combining forms, from *insectum* (insect), meaning *insect*.

in-secti-cide. A substance which kills insects. / in (in) / secare (L. to cut) / caedere (L. to kill).

insulin-...   insulino-...   Combining forms derived from the Latin *insula* (island), in allusion to the islets of Langerhans where insulin is formed.

insulino-gen-ic. Producing insulin. / insula / gen (that which produces) / ic (an adjective-forming suffix).

inter-...   A prefix, derived from the Latin *inter* (between), meaning *among, between, mutually.*

inter-current. Taking place during the course of a previously existing disease (and affecting its progress); occurring in between. / inter (between) / currere (L. to run) / ent (a suffix meaning *that does*).

inter-ject. To introduce between other things. / inter / jacere (L. to throw).

intra-...   A Latin prefix meaning *inside, within.*

intra-nas-al. Inside the nose. / intra / nasus (L. nose) / al (an adjective-forming suffix).

intro-...   A Latin prefix, from *intro* (inwardly), meaning *into, inward, on the inside, within.*

intro-vers-ion. A turning of one's interests inward. / intro / versus (L. a turning) / ion (a Latin noun-forming suffix indicating an *act*).

iod-...   iodi-...   iodino-...   iodo-...   Greek combining forms, from *iodes* (G. violetlike), referring to *iodine, iodides.* *Note:* the reference "violetlike" is an allusion to the violet-colored vapor into which iodine volatilizes.

iodi-metr-y. The determination of the amount of iodine present in a substance. / iodes / metron (G. measure) / y (a noun-forming suffix denoting an *action*).

-ion... A noun-forming suffix, from the Latin *-io*, genit. *-ionis*, denoting *an act, process, condition, state.*

lacerat-ion, A ragged tear of a tissue. / lacerare (L. to tear), past participle, *lacteratus* / ion.

ion-... **iono-**... **ionto-**... Greek combining forms, based on *ion* (going), genit. *iontos*, referring to an *ion.*

ionto-phoresis. The introduction of ions into a tissue. / iontos / phoresis (G. a carrying).

ips-... **ipsi-**... Combining forms, from the Greek *ipsos* (same) and the Latin *ipse* (self), meaning *same, self, one's own.*

ipsi-later-al. Pertaining to, or situated on, the same side. / ipsos / *latus*, genit. *lateris* (a side) / al (an adjective-forming suffix meaning *pertaining to*).

ips-ation. Self-gratification; masturbation. / ipse (self) / ation (a noun-forming suffix denoting an *action*).

ir-... A Latin prefix, having the same function as in- (*no, not, without*), used before a word or combining form beginning with the letter *r*.

ir-revers-ible. That cannot be reversed. / ir / reversus (L. turned backward) / ible (a Latin adjective-forming suffix meaning *able to*).

ir-... **irid-**... **iridi-**... **irido-**... Greek combining forms, from *iris*, genit. *iridos* (rainbow), referring to the *iris of the eye.*

iridi-form. Shaped like the iris of the eye. / iridos / forma (L. shape).

-is-... **-iso-**... Greek combining forms, from *isos* (equal), meaning *equal, same, identical, similar, alike.*

is-auxesis. Equal growth of a part and the whole. / isos / auxesis (G. growth, increase).

isch- ...   **ischo-** ...   Greek combining forms, from *ischein* (to suppress), referring to *stoppage, suppression, deficiency, checking.*

isch-em-ia. A deficiency of blood in a tissue or structure. / ischein / haima (G. blood) / ia (a noun-forming suffix denoting a *disorder*).

ischi- ...   **ischio-** ...   Greek combining forms, from *ischion* (hip), meaning *ischium, hip.*

ischi-alg-ia. Pain in the hip. / ischion / algos (G. pain) / ia (a Latin noun-forming suffix used in names of *diseases*).

-ism ...   A noun-forming suffix, from the Latin *-ismus*, meaning *an act, process, condition, action.*

infant-il-ism. An abnormal retention of infantile characteristics into adult life. / in (not) / fari (L. to speak), fans (present participle), genit. *fantis* / ile (an adjective-forming suffix denoting a characteristic) / ism.

-ismus ...   A noun-forming suffix, from the Latin *-ismus*, denoting *an abnormal condition.*

sphincter-ismus. A spasmodic contraction of a sphincter muscle. / sphinkter (a ringlike muscle surrounding an opening) / ismus.

-ist ...   A noun-forming suffix, from the Latin *-ista*, denoting *a person engaged in a specified occupation, person skilled or learned in a given field.*

ortho-ped-ist. A practitioner of orthopedics. / orthos (G. straight) / pais (G. child), genit. *paidos* / ist.

isthm- ...   **isthmo-** ...   Greek combining forms, from *isthmos* (narrow passage), meaning *isthmus, connecting structure.*

isthm-ec-tom-y. Surgical removal of an isthmus, especially that of the thyroid gland. / isthmos / ek (G. out) / tomos (G. a cut) / y (a suffix denoting an *action*).

ithy-...   ithyo-...   Greek combining forms, from *ithys* (straight), meaning *straight, unbent.*

ithyo-kyphosis. Kyphosis not associated with a lateral curvature. / ithys / kyphosis (G. condition of being humpbacked).

-itic...   An adjective-forming suffix, from the Latin *-iticus*, meaning *caused by, of the nature of, affected with.*

syphil-itic. Affected with syphilis. / siphlos (G. crippled, syphilis) / itic.

-itious...   An adjective-forming suffic, from the Latin *-itius*, meaning *characterized by, of the nature of, having a specified quality.*

icter-itious. Having a jaundiced appearance. / ikteros (G. jaundice) / itious.

-itis...   -itides...   Greek combining forms, from *itis*, plural *itides* (inflammation), meaning *inflammation.*

nephr-itides. The various forms of nephritis, collectively. / nephros (G. kidney) / itides.

-ity...   A noun-forming suffix, from the Latin *-itas*, denoting *a condition, state, character.*

steril-ity. The condition of being sterile. / sterilis (L. barren) / ity.

-ive...   An adjective-forming suffix, from the Latin *-ivus*, meaning *pertaining to, tending to, having the quality of.*

suppurat-ive. Tending to cause suppuration. / suppurare (L. to suppurate), past participle *suppuratus* / ive.

-ization ...   A noun-forming suffix, from the Latin *-izare* and *-ationis,* denoting *a process, act, result, condition.*

fertil-ization. Impregnation; the fusion of an ovum and a spermatozoon. / fertilis (L. fertile) / ization.

-ize ...   A verb-forming suffix, from the Latin *-izare,* meaning *become, cause to be, treat with, subject to, combine with.*

steril-ize. To deprive of reproductive power. / sterilis (L. barren) / ize.

J

jejun- ... **jejuno-** ... Latin combining forms, from *jejunum* (empty), referring to the *jejunum, second part of small intestine. Note:* it was formerly thought that the jejunum is invariably empty after death.

jejuno-stom-y. The formation of an artificial opening in the wall of the jejunum. / jejunum / stoma (G. a mouth, opening) / y (a noun-forming suffix denoting an *action*).

jug- ... A Latin combining form, from *jugare* (to bind together) and *jugum* (a yoke), referring to a *junction, connecting structure.*

con-jug-al. Pertaining to marriage. / con (together) / jugare (L. to join, bind together) / al (an adjective-forming suffix meaning *pertaining to*).

jugul- ... A Latin combining form, from *jugulum* (neck), meaning *neck, throat.*

jugul-ar. Pertaining to, or situated in, the neck. / jugulum / ar (an adjective-forming suffix).

junct- ... A Latin combining form, from *jungere*, past participle *junctus* (to join), meaning *join, unite.*

con-junct-iva. The membrane covering the front part of the eyeball. / con (with, together) / junctus / iva (a suffix denoting a condition, function). *Note:* the conjunctiva was formerly known as the *membrana conjunctiva,* connected membrane (to the eyeball).

juxta- ...   A Latin prefix, from *juxta* (near), meaning *near, beside, close to.*

juxta-glomerul-ar. Situated near a glomerulus. / juxta / glomerulus (L. small ball) / ar (an adjective-forming suffix).

K

kal-... **kali-**... **kalio-**... Latin combining forms, from *kalium* (potassium), meaning *potassium*.

kali-ur-esis. The elimination of potassium in the urine; the passage of urine containing potassium. / kalium / ouron (G. urine) / esis (a Greek suffix denoting a *process*).

kary-... **karyo-**... Greek combining forms, from *karyon* (nut), referring to a *nucleus, kernel, nut*.

karyo-cyte. A nucleated cell. / karyon / kytos (G. a cell).

kata-... A combining form, derived from the Greek *kata* (down), meaning *down, downward*.

kata-phren-ia. A downward trend of the mood. / kata (downward) / phren (G. mind) / ia (a Latin noun-forming suffix used in names of *disorders*).

-kerat-... **kerati-**... **kerato-**... Combining forms, derived from the Greek *keras,* genit. *keratos* (cornea), referring to the *cornea of the eye*.

kerato-centesis. Surgical puncture of the cornea. / keratos (of the cornea) / kentesis (G. a puncture).

kerat-... **kerato-**... Greek combining forms, from *keras,* genit. *keratos* (horn), referring to *horny tissue*.

kerat-in. The tough protein of hair and nails. / keras, keratos / in (a suffix denoting a *protein*).

kerauno-... A Greek combining form, from *keraunos* (lightning), referring to *lightning*.

kerauno-phob-ia. Abnormal fear of lightning. / keraunos / phobos (G. fear) / ia (a noun-forming suffix used in names of *disorders*).

keto-... keton-... Greek combining forms, from *keton* (based on French *acetone*), referring to *ketone*.

keto-lysis. The splitting of ketones. / keton / lysis (G. a breaking up).

kilo-... A Greek prefix, from *chilioi* (thousand), meaning *thousand, thousand times*.

kilo-cycle. A frequency equal to a thousand cycles per second. / chilioi / kyklos (G. circle, cycle).

-kin-... kine-... kinemat-... kines-... kinesio-... kineto-... kino-... Greek combining forms, from *kinema*, genit. *kinematos* (motion), *kinesis* (movement), and *kinetos* (movable), meaning *movement, motion, movable*.

kine-scope. An instrument for measuring the refraction of the eye. / kinema / skopein (G. to examine).

kinesio-logy. The study of motion of living organisms. / kinesis / logy (a Greek suffix indicating a *study*).

klept-... klepti-... klepto-... Greek combining forms, from *kleptein* (to steal), referring to *theft, stealing*.

klept-a-mnes-ia. A defense mechanism by which an act of theft is forgotten. / kleptein / a (without) / mnesis (G. remembrance) / ia (a noun-forming suffix used in names of *disorders*).

koil-... koilo-... Greek combining forms, from *koilos* (hollow), meaning *hollow, concave*.

koil-onych-ia. The condition of having concave nails. / koilos / onyx, onychos (G. nail) / ia (a Latin noun-forming suffix used in names of *disorders*).

kyph- ... **kypho-** ... **kyphot-** ... Greek combining forms, from *kyphos* (hunched, humpbacked), referring to *kyphosis, humpback*.

kyph-osis. The condition of having a humped back. / kyphos / osis (a Greek suffix denoting a *disorder*).

kyphot-ic. Marked by kyphosis. / kyphos / ic (an adjective-forming suffix meaning *marked by*).

kysth- ... **kystho-** ... Greek combining forms, from *kysthos* (vagina), referring to the *vagina*.

kysth-odyn-ia. Pain in the vagina. / kysthos / odyne (G. pain) / ia (a noun-forming suffix used in naming *disorders*).

L

-lab-... -labi-... labio-...   Latin combining forms, from *labium* (lip), referring to a *lip* or *liplike* structure.

labio-plast-y. A plastic operation on a lip. / labium / plastos (G. formed) / y (a noun-forming suffix used to indicate *action*).

lacrim-... lacrima-... lacrimo-...   Latin combining forms, from *lacrima* (a tear), referring to *tears, lacrimal apparatus.*

lacrim-ation. Discharge of tears, especially excessive. / lacrima / ation (a Latin noun-forming suffix denoting an *act*).

lact-... lacti-... lacto-...   Latin combining forms, from *lac*, genit. *lactis* (milk), meaning *milk*.

lacti-vor-ous. Subsisting on milk. / lactis / vorare (L. to devour) / ous (an adjective-forming suffix).

-lal-... lali-... lalo-...   Greek combining forms, from *lalein* (to speak), referring to *speech, speech organs, babble.*

lalo-pleg-ia. Paralysis of the speech organs. / lalein / plege (G. a stroke) / ia (a noun-forming suffix used in names of *diseases*).

-lamell-... lamelli-...   Latin combining forms, from *lamella* (diminutive of *lamina*, a small plate), referring to a *thin plate, scale, layer, lamella.*

97

lamell-ate. Consisting of lamellae. / lamella / ate (a Latin adjective-forming suffix meaning *characterized by*).

lamin-...   lamina-...   lamino-...   Latin combining forms, from *lamina* (thin plate), referring to a *lamina, thin plate, layer.*

lamina-graph-y. Sectional roentgenography. / lamina / graphein (G. to write) / y (a noun-forming suffix denoting an *action*).

lapar-...   laparo-...   Combining forms from the Greek *lapara* (flank), meaning *loin, flank, abdominal wall, abdomen.*

laparo-scop-y. Inspection of the interior of the abdomen. / lapara / skopein (G. examine) / y (a noun-forming suffix denoting an *action*).

laryng-...   laryngo-...   Greek combining forms, from *larynx*, genit. *laryngos* (larynx, voice organ), referring to the *larynx.*

laryngo-scop-y. Inspection of the larynx. / larynx, laryngos / skopein (G. to see) / y (a noun-forming suffix indicating an *action*).

-later-...   latero-...   Latin combining forms, from *latus* (a side), genit. *lateris,* meaning *side, sideways.*

latero-flex-ion. A flexion or bending to the side. / lateris / flectere, past participle *flexus* (to flex) / ion (a noun-forming suffix denoting an *act*).

lecith-...   lecitho-...   Greek combining forms, from *lekithos* (yolk), referring to the *yolk of an egg.*

lecith-al. Pertaining to the yolk of an egg. / lekithos / al (an adjective-forming suffix meaning *pertaining to*).

leio-...   A Greek combining form, from *leios* (smooth), meaning *smooth, glossy, unwrinkled.*

leio-derm-ia. Abnormal smoothness of the skin. / leios / derma (G. skin) / ia (a noun-forming suffix denoting an *abnormal condition*).

lens-... lent-... lenti-... lento-... lenticul-... Latin combining forms, from *lens* (a lentil), genit. *lentis,* diminutive *lenticula,* referring to a *lens,* especially the *crystalline lens of the eye.*

lenti-conus. An abnormal protrusion on the surface of the crystalline lens. / lentis / conus (L. a cone). *Note:* the name "lens," based on "lentil," is an allusion to its shape, which resembles that of a lentil.

lepid-... lepido-... lepo-... Greek combining forms, from *lepis,* genit. *lepidos* (a scale), meaning *scale, flake, husk.*

lepo-thrix. A disorder of hair marked by scaliness. / lepis / thrix (G. hair).

lepr-... lepra-... lepro-... Greek combining forms, from *lepra* (leprosy), meaning *leprosy.*

lepr-oma. A typical lesion of leprosy. / lepra / oma (G. swelling, tumor).

lept-... lepto-... Greek combining forms, from *leptos* (slender), meaning *slender, delicate, thin, narrow.*

lepto-pell-ic. Having a narrow pelvis. / leptos / pellis (G. pelvis) / ic (an adjective-forming suffix meaning *having, marked by*).

lesb-... lesbi-... lesbio-... lesbo-... Greek combining forms, from *Lesbos* (an island in the Aegean where Sappho and her followers flourished), referring to a *lesbian, female homosexual.*

lesbo-gnomon-ic. Indicative of female homosexuality. / Lesbos / gnomon (G. one who knows) / ic (an adjective-forming suffix).

leuc-... **leuco-...** Greek combining forms, from *leukos* (white), referring to *whiteness.*

leuc-in-ur-ia. The presence of leucine in the urine. / leukos / in (a particle used as a suffix to designate certain chemical compounds) / ouron (G. urine) / ia (a noun-forming suffix used in names of *disorders*).

leucocyt-... **leukocyt-...** **leukocyto-...** Greek combining forms, from *leukos* (white) and *kytos* (cell), referring to a *white blood cell, leukocyte.*

leukocyt-ur-ia. The presence of leukocytes in the urine. / leukos / kytos / ouron (G. urine) / ia (a noun-forming suffix used in names of *disorders*).

leuk-... **leuko-...** Greek combining forms, from *leukos* (white), referring to *white blood cells, whiteness.*

leuko-pen-ia. A decrease in the number of white blood cells. / leukos / penesthai (G. to be poor) / ia (a noun-forming suffix used to denote a *disorder*).

levo-... **levul-...** Latin combining forms, from *laevus* (left), meaning *left, on the left side, to the left.*

levo-duc-tion. A turning of the eye to the left. / laevus / ducere (L. to lead) / tion (a Latin noun-forming suffix denoting an *act*).

libid-... **libidin-...** **libido-...** Latin combining forms, from *libido* (pleasure) and *libidinosus* (lusty), referring to *libido, lust, sexual desire.*

libid-a-gnos-ia. The condition of being unaware of the influence of the libido upon one's actions. / libido / a (without) / gnosis (G. knowledge) / ia (a noun-forming suffix used in names of *disorders*).

-lien-... **lieno-...** Latin combining forms, from *lien* (the spleen), referring to the *spleen.*

lien-ec-tom-y. Surgical excision of the spleen. / lien / ek (out) / tome (G. a cutting) / y (a noun-forming suffix denoting an *action*).

ligament-... **ligamento-**... Latin combining forms, from *ligamentum* (binder), meaning *ligament*.

ligamento-pex-y. Surgical fixation of a ligament. / ligamentum / pexis (G. a making secure) / y (a noun-forming suffix denoting an *action*).

lign-... **ligni-**... **ligno-**... Latin combining forms, from *lignum* (wood), meaning *wood*.

lign-eous. Having a woody texture. / lignum / eous (an adjective-forming suffix meaning *like*).

lim-... **limos-**... Greek combining forms, from *limos* (hunger), referring to *hunger, starvation*.

lim-a-sthen-ia. Lack of strength due to hunger. / limos / a (without) / sthenos (G. strength) / ia (a noun-forming suffix denoting a disorder).

-ling-... **lingui-**... Latin combining forms, from *lingua* (tongue), referring to the *tongue*.

sub-lingu-al. Under the tongue. / sub (a prefix meaning beneath) / lingua / al (an adjective-forming suffix denoting a *place*).

lip-... **liparo-**... **lipo-**... Greek combining forms, from *lipos* (fat) and *liparos* (oily, fatty), referring to *fat, oil*.

liparo-cele. A hernia containing a mass of fat. / liparos / kele (G. hernia, rupture).

lique-... **liqui-**... **liquid-**... Latin combining forms, from *liquere* (to be liquid) and *liquidus* (liquid), referring to a *liquid, fluid*.

lique-facient. Causing to become a liquid. / liquere / facient (L. *facere*, to make, present participle *faciens*, genitive *facientis*).

lith-... **litho-**...   Greek combining forms, from *lithos* (stone), referring to a *calculus, concretion, stone.*

litho-trit-y. The act of crushing a calculus. / lithos / terere, past participle *tritus* (to rub, crush) / y (a noun-forming suffix denoting an *action*).

-lob-... **lobo-**...   Latin combining forms, from *lobus* (a lobe), referring to a *lobe, subdivision, projecting part.*

lobo-tom-y. A surgical cut into a lobe. / lobus / tome (G. a cutting) / y (a noun-forming suffix denoting an *action*).

-lobul-...   A Latin combining form, from *lobulus* (a small lobe), referring to a *lobule.*

lobul-ose. Composed of lobules. / lobulus / ose (Latin suffix meaning *full of*).

log-... **logo-**...   Greek combining forms, from *logos* (word), meaning *word, speech, discourse.*

logo-mania. Excessive talkativeness. / logos / mania (G. madness, from *mainesthai*, to rage).

-logy...   Greek suffix, from *logos* (word, study), meaning *science of, study of, branch of knowledge.*

endo-crino-logy. The science of endocrine glands and their products. / endon (G. within) / krinein (G. separate, secrete) / logos.

long-... **longi-**...   Latin combining forms, from *longus* (long), meaning *long, lasting, durable.*

long-ev-ity. Condition of living long. / longus / aevum (L. age) / ity (a Latin suffix forming nouns indicating a *condition*).

loph-... **lophi-**... **lophio-**... **lopho-**...   Combining forms, derived from the Greek *lophos* (ridge), referring to a *tuft, ridge, crest.*

loph-odont. Having ridged molars. / lophos (ridge) / odous, genit. odontos (G. a tooth).

-luc-...   luci-...   Latin combining forms, from *lux* (light), genit. *lucis, lucere* (to shine), referring to *light, illumination.*

trans-luc-ent. Partially transparent. / trans (L. through) / lucere / ent (a Latin adjective-forming suffix meaning *that shows*).

lumb-...   lumbar-...   lumbo-...   Latin combining forms, from *lumbus* (loin) and *lumbaris* (pertaining to the loin), meaning *loin, lumbar.*

lumbo-cost-al. Pertaining to the loin and the ribs. / lumbus / costa (L. rib) / al (an adjective-forming suffix).

lumbri-...   lumbric-...   Combining forms, derived from the Latin *lumbricus* (earthworm), denoting a relationship to *worms, earthworms, roundworms.*

lumbric-osis. The condition of being infested with worms. / lumbricus (worm) / osis (a Greek noun-forming suffix denoting a *disorder, condition*).

lumi-...   lumin-...   lumini-...   lumino-...   Latin combining forms, from *lumen*, genit. *luminis* (light), meaning *light, illumination.*

lumin-escence. The process of giving off light without appreciable heat. / luminis / escentia (L. a noun-forming suffix denoting a *process*).

lun-...   lunat-...   lunato-...   Latin combining forms, from *luna* (moon) and *lunaticus* (moon-struck), referring to *insanity, mental derangement.*

lunato-phob-ia. Fear of insanity. / lunaticus / phobos (G. fear) / ia (a Latin noun-forming suffix used in names of *diseases*).

lun- ...   **luni-** ...   Latin combining forms, from *luna* (the moon), referring to the *moon.*

luna-cy. A mental disorder, formerly assumed to be caused by the moon. / luna / cy (a noun-forming suffix denoting a *condition*).

lute- ...   **lutein-** ...   Combining forms, derived from the Latin *luteus* (yellow), referring to the *corpus luteum.*

lutein-ization. The formation of a corpus luteum. / luteus (yellow) / ization (a Latin noun-forming suffix denoting a *process*).

-lymph- ...   **lymphat-** ...   **lymphati-** ...   **lymphato-** ...   Latin combining forms, from *lympha* (clear water) and *lymphaticus* (pertaining to *lympha*), referring to *lymph, lymphatic system.*

lympho-cyte. A kind of cell found in the blood. / lympha / kytos (G. cell).

lymphaden- ...   **lymphadeno-** ...   Combining forms, derived from the Latin *lympha* (clear water, lymph) and the Greek *aden* (gland), referring to *lymph nodes.*

lymph-adeno-path-y. Any disease of lymph nodes. / lympha / aden / pathos (G. disease) / y (a noun-forming suffix denoting a condition).

lymphang- ...   **lymphangi-** ...   **lymphangio-** ...   Combining forms, from the Latin *lympha* (clear water, lymph) and the Greek *angeion* (vessel), meaning a *lymph vessel.*

lymph-angi-oma. A tumor of lymph vessles. / lympha / angeion / oma (a Greek suffix meaning *tumor*).

lyo- ...   A Greek combining form, from *lyein* (to dissolve), referring to *solution, dissolving.*

lyo-phil-ic. Dissolving readily. / lyein / philein (G. love, like) /

ic (an adjective-forming suffix designating the possession of a specified *quality*).

-lys-... **lysi-**... **-lysis**... **lyso-**... Combining forms, derived from the Greek *lysis* (a loosening), meaning *dissolution, destruction, dissolving, loosing.*

hemo-lysis. A dissolution of red blood cells. / haima (G. blood) / lysis (dissolution).

lysso-... A Greek combining form, from *lyssa* (madness), referring to *rabies.*

lysso-phob-ia. Abnormal fear of rabies. / lyssa / phobos (G. fear) / ia (a noun-forming suffix used in names of *disorders*).

M

-machy... A Greek terminal combining form, from *mache* (a battle), meaning *contest, struggle, battle*.

logo-machy. A fight about words. / logos (G. word) / machia, mache.

macr-... macro-... Greek combining forms, from *makros* (large), meaning *large, long, enlarged*.

macro-cephal-ous. Having a large head. / makros / kephale (G. head) / ous (an adjective-forming suffix).

mal-... male-... Latin combining forms, from *malus* (bad), meaning *improper, faulty, bad, wrong*.

mal-form-ation. A faulty formation. / malus / forma (L. form, shape) / ation (a Latin noun-forming suffix denoting an *action, process*).

malac-... malaco-... Greek combining forms, from *malakos* (soft), meaning *soft, abnormally soft*.

osteo-malac-ia. A disease marked by a softening of the bones. / osteon (G. bone) / malakos / ia (a noun-forming suffix used in names of *diseases*).

malleo-... A Latin combining form, from *malleus* (a hammer), meaning *malleus, the largest auditory ossicle*.

malleo-tom-y. A surgical cutting of the malleus. / malleus / tome (G. a cutting) / y (a noun-forming suffix indicating an action).

malleol-... **malleoli-**... **malleolo-**... Latin combining forms, from *malleolus* (little hammer), referring to a *malleolus*.

malleolo-tom-y. A surgical cutting into a malleolus. / malleolus / tome (G. a cutting) / y (a noun-forming suffix denoting an *action*).

mamm-... **mamma-**... **mammi-**... **mammo-**... Combining forms, derived from the Latin *mamma* (breast), denoting a reference to the *breast* or *mammary gland*.

mamm-ectom-y. The surgical removal of a breast. / mamma (breast) / ek (G. out) / temnein (G. to cut) / y (a noun-forming suffix).

mammil-... **mammilla-**... **mammillo-**... Latin combining forms, from *mammilla* (small breast, teat), meaning *nipple, nipple-like structure.*

mammill-itis. Inflammation of a nipple. / mammilla / itis (G. inflammation).

-man-... **mani-**... **manu-**... Latin combining forms, from *manus* (hand), meaning *hand,* or *hand-like structure.*

longi-man-ous. Having long hands. / longus (L. long) / manus / ous (an adjective-forming suffix meaning *having*).

-mancy... A Greek combining form, from *manteia* (divination), meaning *divination.*

necro-mancy. The foretelling of the future by alleged communication with the dead. / nekros (G. corpse) / manteia.

mandibul-... **mandibuli-**... **mandibulo-**... Latin combining forms, from *mandibulum* (a jaw), referring to the *mandible, lower jawbone.*

mandibuli-form. Resembling the mandible in shape. / mandibulum / forma (L. shape).

-mania- ...   A Greek combining form, from *mania* (madness), meaning *mania, craving, frenzy, madness.*

pyro-mania. A mania for arson. / pyr (G. fire) / mania.

-mas- ...   **masseter-** ...   **massetero-** ...   Combining forms, derived from the Greek *maseter* (a chewer), meaning to *chew, grind, masticate.*

masseter-odyn-ia. The condition in which chewing is painful. / maseter (chewer) / odyne (G. pain) / ia (a Latin noun-forming suffix used in names of *diseases* and *disorders*).

maschal- ...   **maschalo-** ...   Combining forms, from the Greek *maschale* (armpit), referring to the *axilla, armpit.*

maschal-aden-itis. Inflammation of the lymph nodes in the armpit. / maschal (armpit) / aden (G. gland) / itis (inflammation). *Note:* the lymph nodes were once regarded as glands.

maschal-oncus. A mass or tumor of the axilla. / maschal / onkos (G. a tumor or swelling).

-mascul- ...   **masculin-** ...   **masculo-** ...   Latin combining forms, from *masculus* (male) and *masculinus* (masculine), meaning *male, manly, masculine.*

e-mascul-ate. To deprive of masculinity. / e (out) / masculus / ate (a verb-forming suffix meaning *to make, produce*).

mass- ...   **masso-** ...   Combining forms, from the French *masser* (massage), meaning *massage, rub, knead.*

masso-therapy. Treatment by means of massage. / masser / therapeia (G. treatment).

mast- ...   **masto-** ...   Combining forms, derived from the

Greek *mastos* (breast), denoting an involvement of the *breast* or *mammary gland.*

mast-algia. Pain in a breast. / mastos (breast) / algos (G. pain). *Note:* the suffix *ia* is used to form nouns, as names of *diseases, biological classes,* etc.

mastoid-...   mastoideo-...   mastoido-... Greek combining forms, from *mastoeides* (resembling a breast), referring to the *mastoid process, antrum, or cells.*

mastoideo-centesis. Surgical puncture of the mastoid cells. / mastoeides / kentesis (G. a puncture).

matern-...   materno-...   matri-...   matro-... Latin combining forms, from *mater* (mother), *maternus* (maternal), *matrona* (wife, mother), meaning *mother, motherhood.*

matro-clin-ous. Having characteristics derived from the mother. / matrona / clinare (L. to lean) / ous (a Latin adjective-forming suffix meaning *characterized by*).

-maxill-...   maxillo-... Latin combining forms, from *maxilla* (jawbone), referring to the *maxilla, bone of upper jaw.*

maxill-ec-tom y. Excision of a part of the maxilla. / maxilla / ek (out) / tome (G. a cutting) / y (a noun-forming suffix indicating a *process*).

-maz-...   mazo-... Combining forms, derived from the Greek *mazos* (breast), denoting an involvement of the *breast* or *mammary gland.*

maz-odyn-ia. Pain in a breast. / mazos (breast) / odyne (G. pain) / ia (a noun-forming suffix).

-meat-...   meato-... Latin combining forms, from *meatus* (passage), meaning *opening, meatus, passage*

meato-tom-y. The surgical cutting of a meatus. / meatus / tome (G. a cutting) / y (a noun-forming suffix indicating a *process*).

medi-...   **medio-**...   **mid-**...   Latin combining forms, from *medius* (middle), meaning *middle, medial, mean.*

medi-sect. To divide or cut in the middle or midline. / medius / secare, sectus (L. to cut).

-medull-...   **medulli-**...   **medullo-**...   Latin combining forms, from *medulla* (marrow), referring to the *medulla oblongata, bone marrow, inner substance of an organ.*

medull-itis. Inflammation of bone marrow. / medulla / itis (a suffix denoting *inflammation*).

-medull-...   **medullo-**...   Latin combining forms, from *medulla* (marrow), referring to *bone marrow.*

medull-ization. Formation of marrow. / medulla / ization (a noun-forming suffix indicating a *process*).

meg-...   **mega-**...   Greek prefixes, from *megas* (big), meaning *large, big, a million.*

mega-colon. An abnormally large colon. / megas / kolon (G. large intestine).

mega-hertz. An electrical unit of one million cycles per second. / megas / hertz (after H. R. Hertz, German physicist).

megal-...   **megalo-**...   Greek combining forms, from *megale* (fem. of *megas*, large), meaning *large, great, big, powerful.*

megalo-blast. A large erythroblast. / megale / blastos (G. a bud).

-mel-...   A Greek combining form, from *melos* (limb), referring to a *limb, extremity.*

caco-mel-ia. Congenital deformity of a limb. / kakos (G. bad) / melos / ia (a noun-forming suffix used in names of *disorders*).

melan-...   **melani-**...   **melano-**...   Combining forms, derived from the Greek *melas* (black), meaning *black.*

melan-emia. The presence of a black pigment in the blood. / melas (black) / haima (G. blood) / ia (a noun-forming suffix).

melano-phore. A cell containing melanin, a black pigment. / melas / phoros (G. one who carries). *Note:* the combining form *melan* is based on the genitive form of *melas,* which is *melanos.*

meli-... **melisso-**... **melit-**... Greek combining forms, from *meli,* genit. *melitos* (honey) and *melissa* (a bee), meaning *honey, bee.*

meli-bi-ose. A kind of sugar. / meli / bi (double) / ose (a suffix denoting a sugar).

melisso-phob-ia. Fear of bees. / melissa / phobos (G. fear) / ia (a Latin suffix used to denote a *condition*).

-membran-... **membrani-**... **membrano-**... Latin combining forms, from *membrana* (membrane), referring to a *thin layer of tissue, membrane.*

membran-aceous. Having the nature or structure of a membrane. / membrana / aceous (a Latin adjective-forming suffix meaning *of the nature of*).

-men-... **meno-**... **menstru-**... Combining forms, from the Greek *men,* genit. *menos* (month) and the Latin *menstruatus,* past participle of *menstruare* (menstruato), referring to *menstruation, menses, month.*

menstru-ation. The monthly flow of blood and sloughed-off tissue from the uterus. / menstruare / ation (a Latin noun-forming suffix denoting a *process*).

men-arche. The first menstrual period of a girl at puberty. / men / arche (G. beginning).

mening-... **meninge-**... **meningeo-**... **meningi-**... **meningo-**... Greek combining forms, from *meninx,* genit. *meningos* (membrane), referring to *membranes, meninges.*

meningi-oma. A tumor of the meninges. / meningos / oma
(Greek suffix meaning *tumor*).

-ment- ... **menti-** ... Latin combining forms, from *mens,*
genit. *mentis* (mind), meaning *mind, mental.*

de-ment-ia. A form of mental deterioration. / de (out from) /
mens, mentis (mind) / ia (a Latin noun-forming suffix used in
names of *diseases*).

ment- ... **mento-** ... Combining forms, derived from the
Latin *mentum* (chin), denoting a reference to the *chin* or *lower
jaw.*

mento-labial. Pertaining to the chin and a lip. / mentum (chin)
/ labium (L. lip).

mentul- ... **mentuli-** ... **mentulo-** ... Latin combining
forms, from *mentula* (penis), meaning *penis.*

mentul-agra. Pain in the penis associated with a persistent erec-
tion. / mentula / agra (G. seizure of pain).

mer- ... **meri-** ... **mero-** ... Greek combining forms,
from *meros* (part), meaning *part, segment, fraction.*

meri-spore. A spore produced by the segmentation of another
spore. / meros / spora (G. a seed).

mercur- ... **mercuri-** ... **mercuro-** ... Latin combining
forms, from *mercurius* (mercury), meaning *mercury.*

mercuri-al-ize. To impregnate with mercury. / mercurius / al (a
Latin adjective-forming suffix) / ize (a Latin verb-forming suffix meaning *treat with*).

mes- ... **mesi-** ... **mesio-** ... **meso-** ... Greek combining forms, from *mesos* (middle), meaning *middle, median, intermediate.*

mes-en-cephal-on. The midbrain. / mesos / en (in) / kephale (G.
head) / on (a noun-making suffix).

met-...   meta-...   Prefixes, derived from the Greek *meta* (*after, beside, with, beyond*), having a multiplicity of meanings, such as *changed (in form or place), altered, reversed, with, alongside, beyond, over, on the farther side of, later, after, a derivative of, a modification of.*

meta-morph-osis. A change from one developmental stage to another. / meta (over) / morphe (form) / osis (a Greek noun-forming suffix denoting an *action*).

meta-sta-sis. The transfer of a pathologic condition from one place to another. / meta (after) / histanai (G. to place) / sis (a Greek noun-forming suffix denoting an *activity* or *condition*).

metop-...   metopo-...   Greek combining forms, from *metopon* (forehead), meaning *forehead.*

metop-odyn-ia. Pain in the region of the forehead. / metopon / odyne (G. pain) ia (a Latin noun-forming suffix used in names of *disorders*).

-metr-...   metra-...   metro-...   Greek combining forms, from *metra* (uterus), meaning *uterus.*

metr-ectas-ia. An abnormal dilatation of the uterus. / metra / ektasis (G. a distention) / ia (a noun-forming suffix used in names of diseases).

metr-...   metro-...   -metry...   Greek combining forms, from *metron* (measure), referring to *measure, measurement.*

psycho-metry. Measurement of psychic processes. / psyche (G. soul, spirit) / metry (a Greek suffix indicating the *process of measuring*, from *metron*, measure).

mi-...   mio-...   miot-...   Greek combining forms, from *myein* (to close), meaning *decrease, less, little.*

mi-osis. Abnormal contraction of the pupil. / myein / osis (a noun-forming suffix denoting a *condition*).

micr- ...   **micro-** ...   Greek combining forms, from *mikros* (small), meaning *small, microscopic, one-millionth.*

micr-en-cephal-y. Abnormal smallness of the brain. / mikros / en (in) / kephale (G. head) / y (a noun-forming suffix denoting a *condition*).

milli- ...   A Latin prefix, from *mille* (a thousand), meaning *one thousandth.*

milli-meter. One thousandth part of a meter. / mille / metron (G. measure).

mis- ...   **miso-** ...   Greek combining forms, from *misein* (to hate), referring to *hate, dislike, aversion.*

miso-gam-y. Aversion for marriage. / misein / gamos (G. marriage) / y (a noun-forming suffix denoting a *condition, characteristic.*

mit- ...   **mito-** ...   Greek combining forms, from *mitos* (a thread), meaning *thread, threadlike structure.*

mito-chondria. Rodlike structures occurring in the cytoplasm of most cells. / mitos / chondrion (G. a small piece of cartilage).

-mnem- ...   **mnemon-** ...   **-mnesia** ...   **-mnesis** ...   Greek combining forms, from *mnemon* (mindful) and *mnasthai* (to remember), referring to *memory, remembrance.*

hypo-mnesis. The condition of having a weak memory. / hypo (G. less than) / mnesis (condition of memory), from mnasthai.

mogi- ...   A combining form, derived from the Greek *mogis* (with difficulty), meaning *difficult, laborious, unsuccessful.*

mogi-toc-ia. Difficult childbirth. / mogis (difficult) / tokos (G. birth) / ia (a Latin noun-forming suffix used in names of *diseases* and *disorders*).

mon- ...   **mono-** ...   Greek prefixes, from *monos* (one), meaning *one, single, alone.*

mono-mania. Mental derangement about one subject. / monos / mania (G. madness).

-morph-... **morpho-**... **-morphy**... Greek combining forms, from *morphe* (form), meaning *form, shape, configuration.*

morpho-log-y. The study of forms. / morphe / logos (G. word, study) / y (a noun-forming suffix).

mort-... **morti-**... Combining forms, derived from the Latin *mors*, genit. *mortis* (death), referring to *death, dying.*

mort-ician. A person trained in preparing the dead for burial. / mors (death) / ician (one skilled in some specified field).

-mot-... **moto-**... **motor-**... **motoro-**... Latin combining forms, from *movere*, past participle *motus* (to move), referring to *movement, motion.*

motor-icity. The ability to move or to cause motion. / motus / icity (Latin suffix denoting a *quality*).

-muc-... **muci-**... **mucin-**... **mucino-**... **muco-**... Latin combining forms, from *mucus* (fluid covering mucous membranes), meaning *mucus, mucin.*

muci-fer-ous. Producing or bearing mucus. / mucus / ferre (L. bear, produce) / ous (a Latin adjective-forming suffix).

multi-... A Latin prefix, from *multus* (many), meaning *many, multiple, much.*

multi-fidus. Divided into several parts. / multus / fidus (L. divided).

-mut-... **muta-**... Latin combining forms, from *mutare* (to change), referring to *mutation, transformation, change.*

muta-gen. An agent producing change or mutation. / mutare / gen (a suffix meaning *something that produces*, from the Greek *gignesthai*, to be born).

-my-...   myo-...   Greek combining forms, from *mys*, genit. *myos* (muscle), meaning *muscle, muscle tissue.*

myo-card-ium. The muscular tissue forming the wall of the heart. / myos / kardia (G. heart) / ium (a suffix used to form nouns).

myc-...   mycet-...   myceto-...   myco-...   Greek combining forms, from *mykes*, plural *myketes* (mushroom), referring to a *fungus.*

myc-osis. Any disease caused by a fungus. / mykes / osis (a Greek suffix used to indicate a *disease* or *disorder*).

-mycin...   A Greek terminal combining form, from *mykes* (a fungus) and *in* (a suffix denoting a medicinal preparation), meaning *an antibiotic derived from a fungus.*

strepto-mycin. An antibiotic obtained from *Streptomyces griseus.* / streptos (G. twisted) / mykes / in.

myel-..   myelo-...   Greek combining forms, from *myelos* (marrow), referring to the *spinal cord, bone marrow.*

myelo-cele. A hernia in which the spinal cord forms the protruding mass. / myelos / kele (G. swelling, hernia).

myel-itis. Inflammation of bone marrow. / myelos / itis (a suffix used to denote *inflammation*).

myelin-...   myelino-...   Greek combining forms, from *myelos* (marrow), meaning *myelin, myelin sheath.*

myelin-osis. Any disease or disorder of myelin. / osis (a Greek noun-forming suffix denoting an *abnormal condition*).

myria-...   A Greek prefix, from *myrios* (countless), meaning *very many, numerous, ten thousand.*

myria-pod. Having many legs. / myrias (ten thousand) / pous (G. foot), genit. *podos.*

myring-...   **myringo-**...   Combining forms, derived from the Latin *myringa* (membrane), referring to the *eardrum*.

myring-ectom-y. Surgical excision of the eardrum. / myringa (membrane; eardrum) / ek (G. out) / temnein (G. cut) / y (a noun-forming suffix denoting an action).

myrmeco-...   A Greek combining form, from *myrmex* (ant), genit. *myrmekos*, referring to *ants*.

myrmeco-phagous. Subsisting on ants. / myrmekos / phagein (G. to eat) / ous (an adjective-forming suffix denoting a *characteristic*).

N

nan-... **nani-...** **nano-...** Latin combining forms, from *nanus* (dwarf), indicating *smallness, dwarfishness.*

nano-mel-ous. Having abnormally small limbs. / nanus / melos (G. a limb) / ous (an adjective-forming suffix meaning *characterized by, having*).

nar-... **nari-...** **nario-...** Latin combining forms, from *naris,* plural *nares* (nostril), referring to the *nostrils* or a *nostril.*

intra-nari-al. Situated within a nostril. / intra (L. inside) / naris / al (an adjective-forming suffix).

narco-... **narcot-...** Combining forms, from the Greek *narke* (numbness) and the Latin *narcoticus* (narcotic), referring to *sleep, stupor, lethargy, numbness, insensibility.*

narco-ana-lysis. Psychoanalysis applied to a patient who is under the influence of a narcotic. / narke / ana (throughout) / lysis (G. a releasing).

nas-... **naso-...** Latin combining forms, from *nasus* (nose), meaning *nose.*

naso-labi-al. Pertaining to the nose and the lip. / labium (L. lip) / al (an adjective-forming suffix meaning *pertaining to*).

nat-... **nati-...** **-natia...** Combining forms, from the Latin *nasci* (pp. *natus*), to be born, denoting a relationship to *birth.*

nat-al. Pertaining to or involving birth. / nat / al (L. an adjective-forming suffix meaning *pertaining to*).

pre-nat-al. Occurring before birth. / prae (L. before) / nat / al.

ne- . . .   neo- . . .   Greek combining forms, from *neos* (new), meaning *new, recent, foreign, strange.*

miso-ne-ism. An aversion for new things. / misein (G. to dislike) / neos / ism (a noun-forming suffix indicating a *condition*).

necr- . . .   necro- . . .   necrot- . . .   necroto- . . .   Combining forms, derived from the Greek *nekros* (corpse), referring to *death, dead tissue, dead body.*

necr-ectom-y. The removal or excision of dead tissue. / nekros (corpse) / ek (G. out) / temnein (G. cut) / y (a noun-forming suffix denoting an *action*).

nemat- . . .   nemato- . . .   nematod- . . .   Greek combining forms, from *nema*, genit. *nematos* (thread), referring to *nematodes, parasitic worms.*

nemat-od-iasis. Infestation with nematodes. / nematos / oeides, eidos (shape) / iasis (G. diseased condition).

neph- . . .   nephel- . . .   nephelo- . . .   Greek combining forms from *nephele*, nephos (cloud), referring to *a cloud, turbidity.*

nephelo-meter. An apparatus for measuring the concentration of a substance in a suspension by determining the degree of turbidity. / nephele / meter (a device used for measuring, from the Greek *metron*, measure).

nephr- . . .   nephrit- . . .   nephro- . . .   Greek combining forms, from *nephros* (kidney) and *nephritikos* (of the kidneys), referring to the *kidney.*

nephr-ec-tom-y. Surgical removal of a kidney. / nephros / ek (G. out) / tomos (G. a cut) / y (a noun-forming suffix denoting an *action*).

nerv- ... **nervi-** ... **nervo-** ...   Latin combining forms, from *nervus* (nerve, cord), meaning *nerve, nerve tissue, nervous system.*

nervo-cide. An agent which destroys nerves. / nervus / caedere (to kill, cut down).

neur- ... **neuri-** ... **neuro-** ...   Greek combining forms, from *neuron* (sinew, nerve), meaning *nerve, nerve tissue, nervous system.*

neuro-glia. The supporting structure of the nervous system. / neuron / glia, gloios (G. glue).

neutr- ... **neutro-** ...   Latin combining forms, from *neutralis* (neutral), meaning *neutral, middle position, neither.*

neutro-cyte. A cell stainable by neutral dyes. / neutralis / kytos (G. cell).

nigr- ... **nigri-** ... **nigro-** ...   Latin combining forms, from *nigrescere* (to grow black), referring to *blackness.*

nigr-escence. The process of becoming black. / niger (L. black), nigrescere (to grow black) / escence (a Latin suffix denoting a *process*).

nitr- ... **nitri-** ... **nitrit-** ... **nitro-** ...   Greek combining forms, from *nitron* (niter), referring to *nitrogen, nitrates, nitrites.*

nitrit-oid. Similar to a nitrite. / nitron / oeides (G. resembling).

noci- ...   A Latin combining form, from *nocere* (to hurt), referring to *injury, pain.*

noci-ceptive. Capable of receiving stimuli of pain. / nocere / recipere (L. receive), past participle receptus / ive (a suffix meaning *having the quality of*).

noct- ... **nocti-** ... **nocto-** ...   Latin combining forms, from *nox,* genit. *noctis* (night), meaning *night, darkness.*

noct-albumin-ur-ia. The presence of albumin in the urine produced by the kidneys during the night. / noctis / albumin (L. album, white) / ouron (G. urine) / ia (a noun-forming suffix used in names of *disorders*).

nom- . . .   **nomo-** . . .   Greek combining forms, from *nomos* (law), meaning *law, custom, usage.*

nomo-topic. Occurring in the usual place. / nomos / *topos* (G. a place) / ic (an adjective-forming suffix).

non- . . .   A Latin prefix, from *non* (not), meaning *not, negative.*

non-vi-able. Not capable of surviving. / non / vie (French, life) / able (an adjective-forming suffix meaning *able to*).

norm- . . .   **normal-** . . .   **normo-** . . .   Latin combining forms, from *norma* (a rule) and *normalis* (according to a rule), meaning *normal, conforming to a rule.*

normo-cyte. A normal red blood cell. / norma / kytos (G. cell).

normal-ization. The process of making normal. / normalis / ization (a noun-forming suffix denoting a *process*).

-nos- . . .   **noso-** . . .   Combining forms, derived from the Greek *nosos* (disease), referring to *disease, illness, disorder.*

noso-graph-y. A description of diseases or a particular disease. / nosos (disease) / graphein (G. write, describe) / y (a noun-forming suffix denoting an *action* or the result of an *action*).

not- . . .   **noti-** . . .   **noto-** . . .   Combining forms, derived from the Greek *noton* (the back), referring to the *back of the body* or to a *back part.*

not-odynia. Pain in the back. / not (the back) / odyne (G. pain). *Note:* the suffix *ia* indicates a condition.

noto-chord. The structure which is the primitive skeleton of the spine, in the embryo. / noto / chorde (G. string).

nucle-...   nuclei-...   nucleo-...   Latin combining forms, derived from *nucleus,* a contraction of *nuculeus,* the diminutive of *nux,* genit. *nucis* (a nut), referring to *nucleus, group of nerve cells, central element.*

nuclei-form. Shaped like a nucleus. / nuculeus / forma (L. shape).

nud-...   nudi-...   nudo-...   Latin combining forms, from *nudus* (nude), meaning *nude, bare, uncovered.*

nudi-phob-ia. An aversion for nudity. / nudus / phobos (G. fear, aversion) / ia (a noun-forming suffix used in names of *disorders*).

nulli-...   A Latin form, from *nullus* (none), meaning *none, nothing, no.*

nulli-gravida. A woman who has never been pregnant. / nullus / gravida (L. pregnant).

nutri-...   nutrio-...   Latin combining forms, from *nutrire,* past participle *nutritus* (to nourish), referring to *nutrition, nourishment, food.*

nutri-tion-ist. A person learned in nutrition. / nutrire / tion (a suffix indicating an *act*) / ist (a noun-forming suffix meaning *one who*).

nyct-...   nycti-...   nycto-...   Greek combining forms, from *nyx,* genit. *nyktos* (night), referring to *darkness, night.*

nyct-al-op-ia. The inability to see properly at night. / nyktos / alaos (G. blind) / ops (G. eye) / ia (a noun-forming suffix used in names of *diseases*).

nymph-...   nympho-...   Greek combining forms, from *nymphe* (bride), referring to *sexual desire by a woman* and to a *labium minus.*

nympho-mania. Keen sexual desire felt by a woman. / nymphe / mania (madness).

nymph-ec-tom-y. Surgical excision of the labia minora. / nymphe / ek (G. out) / tome (G. a cutting) / y (a noun-forming suffix denoting an *action*).

nystagm-... nystagmi-... nystagmo-... Greek combining forms, from *nystazein* (to be sleepy or to nod in one's sleep) and *nystagmos* (drowsiness), referring to *nystagmus, nodding*.

nystagmo-genic. Producing nystagmus. / nystagmos / gen (a suffix meaning *that which produces*) / ic (an adjective-forming suffix).

O

ob-... A Latin prefix having a variety of meanings, as *toward, against, over, in front, upon, inversely,* and others.

ob-liter-ate. To destroy; erase. / ob (against) / litera, littera (a letter) / ate (a verb-forming suffix denoting an *action*). *Note:* ob becomes o before the letter *m, oc* before a *c, of* before an *f, op* before a *p.*

oc-... A Latin prefix, regarded as a variant form of *ob,* used before a *c.* See under *ob.*

oc-clude. To close or block a passage. / ob, oc / claudere (L. to close).

occipit-... **occipito-**... Latin combining forms, from *occiput* (back of skull) and *occipitalis* (pertaining to the occiput), referring to the *occiput.*

occipito-ment-al. Pertaining to the occiput and the chin. / occipitalis / mentum (L. chin) / al (an adjective-forming suffix meaning *pertaining to*).

ochro-... A Greek combining form, from *ochros* (pale yellow), referring to the color *pale yellow.*

ochro-derm-ia. An abnormal condition in which the skin is pale yellow. / ochros / derma (G. skin) / ia (a noun-forming suffix used to denote a *disorder*).

124

oct-... octa-... octi-... octo-... Combining forms, derived from the Greek *okto* (eight), meaning *eight, eight times.*

octi-para. A woman who has borne eight children in separate pregnancies. / okto (eight) / parere (L. to bring forth).

-ocul-... oculi-... oculo-... Latin combining forms, from *oculus* (eye), referring to the *eye, eyeball.*

oculo-motor. Pertaining to the movements of the eyeball. / oculus / movere (L. to move, past participle *motus*).

-ode... odo-... Greek combining forms, from *hodos* (way, path), meaning *way, path.*

an-ode. The positively charged electrode of a battery. / ana (G. up) / hodos.

odo-meter. An instrument for measuring distances traveled by a vehicle. / hodos / meter (something that measures, from *metron*, G. measure, and *er*, a suffix denoting a thing performing a specified *function*).

odont-... odontin-... -odontia... -odontics... odontist ... odonto-... Greek combining forms, from *odon* (tooth), genit. *odontos*, referring to *teeth, dentists, dentistry.*

odonto-scope. A small mirror used by dentists for inspecting the teeth. / odontos / scope (an instrument for visual inspection, from the Greek *skopein*, to inspect).

orth-odont-ia. The branch of dentistry dealing with irregularities of teeth. / orthos (G. straight) / odontos / ia (a noun-forming suffix used to denote a *practice*).

odori-... odoro-... Latin combining forms, from *odor* (odor), meaning *odor, aroma, fragrance.*

odori-fer-ous. Having or bearing an odor. / odor / ferre (L. bear) / ous (an adjective-forming suffix meaning *having*).

-odyn- ...   **odyno-** ...   **-odynia** ...   Greek combining forms, from *odyne* (pain), meaning *pain, ache, discomfort*.

odyn-acusis. A condition in which moderate sounds cause pain in the ears. / odyne / akousis (G. hearing).

of- ...   A Latin prefix, a variant of *ob*, used before an *f*. See under *ob*.

of-fer-ing. Something that is offered, as a sacrifice. / ob, of (before) / ferre (L. to bring) / ing (a noun-forming suffix).

ole- ...   **oleo-** ...   Latin combining forms, from *oleum* (oil), meaning *oil*.

oleo-therapy. Treatment of disease with oil. / oleum / therapeia (G. treatment).

olecran- ...   **olecrano-** ...   Greek combining forms, from *olekranon* (olecranon, "head of elbow"), referring to the *olecranon*.

olecrano-humer-al. Pertaining to the olecranon and the humerus. / olekranon / humerus (L. upper arm, bone of upper arm) / al (an adjective-forming suffix).

olecranarthr- ...   **olecranarthro-** ...   Combining forms, derived from the Greek *olene* (elbow), *kranion* (head), arthron (joint), referring to the *elbow, elbow joint*.

olecranarthr-itis. Inflammation or arthritis of the elbow joint. / olene (elbow) / kranion (head) / arthron (joint) / itis (a Greek suffix denoting *inflammation*).

olfact- ...   **olfacti-** ...   **olfacto-** ...   Latin combining forms, from *olfacere* (to smell), past participle *olfactus*, meaning *smell, sense of smell, act of smelling, odor*.

olfacto-phob-ia. An aversion for or fear of certain odors. / olfactus / phobos (G. fear) / ia (a noun-forming suffix denoting an *abnormal condition*).

-olig- ... **oligo-** ... Greek combining forms, from *oligos* (small), meaning *few, little, scanty, deficient, insufficient.*

oligo-meno-rrhea. Scanty menstruation. / oligos / men (G. month) / rheein (G. to flow). *Note:* doubling of the *r* in *rrhea* is explained under *chylorrhea.*

om- ... **oma-** ... **omo** ... Greek combining forms, from *omos* (shoulder), referring to the *shoulder.*

om-alg-ia. Pain in the shoulder. / omos / algos (G. pain) / ia (a noun-forming suffix used in names of *diseases*).

-oma ... *plural* **-omas** ... *plural* **-omata** ... Greek terminal combining forms, from *oma* (a tumor), genit. *omatos*, referring to a *tumor, mass, growth.*

ele-oma. A tumor composed of oil that has been injected into a tissue. / elaion (G. oil) / oma.

omarthr- ... **omartho-** ... Greek combining forms, from *omos* (shoulder) and *arthron* (joint), referring to the *shoulder joint.*

om-arthro-tom-y. A surgical incision into the shoulder joint. / omos / arthron / tome (G. a cutting) / y (a noun-forming suffix indicating an *action*).

oment- ... **omenti-** ... **omento-** ... Latin combining forms, from *omentum* (omentum), referring to the *omentum majus* and *omentum minus.*

omento-pex-y. The attachment of the omentum to another tissue or organ. / omentum / pexis (G. a making secure) / y (a noun-making suffix denoting an *action*).

omni- ... A prefix derived from the Latin *omnis* (all), meaning *everywhere, unrestricted, universal, all.*

omni-potent. Unlimited in power or authority. / omni (unrestricted) / potentia (L. power).

omni-vor-ous. Eating both animal and vegetable food; devouring all kinds of food. / omni (all) / vorare (L. to devour) / ous (an adjective-forming suffix).

omphal- . . .   **omphali-** . . .   **omphalo-** . . .   Greek combining forms, from *omphalos* (navel), meaning *navel.*

omphalo-cele. A herniation of the navel. / omphalos / kele (G. hernia).

onco- . . .   A Greek combining form, from onkos (mass, tumor), referring to a *tumor, mass, growth.*

onco-logy. The study of tumors. / onkos / logia (a study, from the Greek *logos,* word, study).

oneir- . . .   **oneiro-** . . .   Combining forms, derived from the Greek *oneiros* (dream), referring to *dreams.*

oneiro-scop-y. Diagnosis of a mental condition by the analysis of the patient's dreams. / oneiros (dream) / skopein (G. to examine) / y (a noun-forming suffix denoting an *action*).

onomato- . . .   A Greek combining form, from *onoma,* genit. *onomatos,* meaning *name, word, term, nomenclature.*

onomato-phob-ia. Fear of certain words or names. / onomatos / phobos (G. fear) / ia (a noun-forming suffix used in names of *disorders*).

onto- . . .   A Greek combining form, from *einai* (to be), present participle *on,* genit. *ontos,* denoting *being, existence, organism.*

onto-geny. The development of an individual organism. / ontos / geneia (G. development).

-onych- . . .   **onycho-** . . .   Greek combining forms, from *onyx,* genit. *onychos,* meaning *nail, claw.*

onycho-malac-ia. Abnormal softening of the nails. / onychos /

malakos (G. soft) / ia (a noun-forming suffix used in names of *disorders*).

-onym-... **-onymy**... Greek combining forms, from *onyma* (name), referring to *name, title, nomenclature*.

top-onym. The name of a region, as of the body. / topos (G. a region) / onyma.

oo-... A combining form, derived from the Greek *oon* (an egg), referring to an *ovum, egg, female reproductive cell*.

oo-genesis. The development of an ovum. / oon (egg) / genesis (G. origin, development).

oophor-... **oophoro-**... Greek combining forms, from *oon* (an egg) and *pherein* (to bear), referring to the ovary.

oophor-ec-tom-y. The surgical excision of an ovary. / oon / pherein / ek (G. out) / tome (G. a cutting) / y (a suffix indicating an *action*).

op-... A Latin prefix, a variant of *ob*, used before a *p*. See under *ob*.

op-pilat-ive. Something that tends to constipate. / ob, op / oppilare (L. to stop up), past participle *oppilatus* / ive (a noun-forming suffix denoting a *tendency*).

-op-... **-ops-**... **-opsis**... Greek combining forms, from *ops* (eye) and *opsis* (sight), referring to *sight, vision*.

cyan-op-ia. A disorder in which all objects appear blue. / kyanos (blue) / opsis (sight) / ia (a noun-forming suffix denoting a *disorder*).

stere-opsis. Vision in three dimensions. / stereos (hard, three-dimensional) / opsis (sight, vision).

ophid-... **ophidio-**... Greek combining forms, from *ophis* (snake, serpent) and *ophidion* (a small snake or serpent), meaning *snake, serpent*.

ophidio-phob-ia. Excessive fear of snakes. / ophidion / phobos (G. fear) / ia (a noun-forming suffix denoting an *abnormal condition*).

-ophthalm- ... **ophthalmo-** ... Greek combining forms, from *ophthalmos* (eye), referring to the *eye, eyeball.*

ophthalmo-pleg-ia. Paralysis of the muscles of the eye. / ophthalmos / plege (G. stroke) / ia (a Latin noun-forming suffix used in names of *diseases*).

-opia ... A Greek suffix, from *ops* (eye) and *ia* (a suffix denoting a disorder), referring to a *visual defect, eye defect.*

presby-op-ia. Progressive farsightedness associated with aging. / presbys (G. old) / ops / ia.

opisth- ... **opistho-** ... Combining forms, derived from the Greek *opisthen* (behind), meaning *in the back, backward, behind.*

opistho-gnath-ous. Having receding jaws. / opistho (backward) / gnathos (G. jaw) / ous (an adjective-forming suffix).

opisth-enar. The back of the hand. / opisth / thenar (G. palm of the hand).

opsino- ... **opson-** ... **opsoni-** ... **opsono-** ... Greek combining forms, from *opsonion* (food), meaning *opsonin.*

opson-ize. To make bacteria more susceptible to destruction by phagocytes. / opsonion / ize (a verb-forming suffix meaning *cause to be*).

optic- ... **optico-** ... Greek combining forms, from *optikos* (pertaining to sight), referring to *optics, optic nerve, eyes, sight.*

optico-kinetic. Pertaining to movement of the eyes. / optikos / kinetikos (G. causing motion).

opto- ... A Greek prefix, from *optos* (visible, seen), referring to *vision, eye.*

opto-gram. The image of an object on the retina. / optos / gram (a suffix meaning something *written* or otherwise *recorded,* from the Greek *gramma,* writing).

-or- ...   **oro-** ...   Latin combining forms, from *os,* genit. *oris* (mouth), meaning *mouth, opening.*

peri-or-al. Surrounding the mouth. / peri (G. around) / oris / al (an adjective-forming suffix).

-or ...   A noun-forming suffix, from the Latin *-or,* denoting *a person or thing performing a specified function, a condition, quality.*

respirat-or. An apparatus used to administer artificial respiration. / respirare (L. respire), past participle *respiratus* / or.

pall-or. The condition of being pale. / pallere (L. to be pale) / or.

orbit- ...   **orbito-** ...   Latin combining forms, from *orbita* (path), referring to the *orbit, eye socket.*

orbito-tom-y. A surgical cutting into an orbit. / orbita / tome (G. a cutting) / y (a noun-forming suffix indicating an *action*).

orch- ...   **orchi-** ...   **orchid-** ...   **orchido-** ...   **orchio-** ...   Greek combining forms, from *orchis* (testis), denoting a *testicle. Note: orchid* is based on *orchidis,* a faulty genitive of the Latin *orchis; orchido* is based on *orchidos,* a form mistaken as the genitive of the Greek *orchis.*

orchido-tom-y. A surgical cutting into a testicle. / orchidos (see note above) / tome (G. a cutting) / y (a noun-forming suffix denoting an *action*).

-orex- ...   **orexi** ...   Combining forms, from the Greek *orexis* (appetite), referring to *appetite for food, desire, striving.*

an-orex-ia. A lack of appetite for food. / an (a prefix indicating negativity or absence of) / orex (appetite) / ia (a noun-forming suffix indicating a condition).

orexi-fugic. Diminishing or suppressing the appetite. / orexi (appetite) / fugere (L. to flee).

organ-...   organo-...   Greek combining forms, from *organon* (organ), meaning *organ*.

organo-therapy. Treatment with animal organs or organ extracts. / organon / therapeia (G. treatment).

ornith-...   ornitho-...   Combining forms, from the Greek *ornis,* genit. *ornithos* (a bird), denoting a relationship to *birds*.

ornitho-logy. The branch of science dealing with birds. / ornitho / logos (G. a treatise concerning a given subject).

ornitho-phobia. An abnormal fear of birds. / ornitho / phobos (G. fear).

oro-...   A Greek combining form, from *oros* (mountain), meaning *mountain*.

oro-geny. The formation of mountains. / oros / geneia (development), from the Greek *gignesthai* (be born).

orrho-...   A Greek combining form, from *orrhos* (whey), meaning *serum*.

orrho-log-y. The science dealing with the properties and uses of serums. / orrhos / logos (G. word, study) / y (a noun-forming suffix denoting an *action, pursuit*).

orth-...   ortho-...   Greek combining forms, from *orthos* (straight), meaning *correct, normal, straight*.

ortho-paed-ics. The branch of surgery dealing with bones, joints, and related structures. / orthos / pais, genit. paidos (G. child) / ics (a noun-forming suffix referring to a *science, study*).

-ory...   1. An adjective-forming suffix, from the Latin *-orius,* meaning *of, having the nature of, pertaining to, serving for.* 2.

A noun-forming suffix meaning *a place for, a thing for, that which serves for.*

incis-ory. Suitable or used for cutting. / incidere (L. to cut) / ory.

cremat-ory. A place where dead bodies are cremated. / cremare (L. to burn to ashes), past participle *crematus* / ory.

osche- ... **oscheo-** ...   Greek combining forms, from *oscheon* (scrotum), referring to the *scrotum.*

osche-oma. A tumor of the scrotum. / oscheon / oma (G. swelling, tumor).

oscill- ... **oscillo-** ...   Latin combining forms, from *oscillare* (to swing), meaning *oscillate, fluctuate, swing.*

oscillo-graph. An instrument used to record variations in electrical potential or currents. / oscillare / graphein (G. to write, record).

-ose ...   1. An adjective-forming suffix, from the Latin *-osus,* meaning *provided with, having, like.* 2. A noun-forming suffix denoting *a sugar, carbohydrate, product of protein hydrolysis.*

ram-ose. Provided with branches. / ramus (L. branch) / ose.

sucr-ose. A disaccharide sugar obtained from sugar cane, maple, etc. / sucre (Fr. sugar) / ose.

-osis ...   A noun-forming suffix, from the Greek *-osis,* denoting *an action, condition, abnormal condition, disorder, disease.*

a-vit-amin-osis. An abnormal condition resulting from an insufficiency of vitamins in the diet. / a (without) / vita (L. life) / amine (a chemical compound derived from ammonia) / osis.

-osm- ... **osmio-** ... **osmo-** ...   Greek combining forms, from *osme* (odor), referring to *smell, odor.*

osmo-lagn-ia. Sexual desire stimulated or aroused by certain odors. / osme / lagneia (G. lust) / ia (a noun-forming suffix denoting a *condition*).

osmo- ...   **osmoso-** ...   Greek combining forms, from *osmos* (impulse), meaning *osmosis*.

osmo-philic. Designating a solution which is subject to osmosis. / osmos / philein (G. to love) / ic (an adjective-forming suffix meaning *characterized by*).

-osphresia ...   **osphresio-** ...   Greek combining forms, from *osphresis* (sense of smell), referring to *smell, sense of smell*.

oxy-osphres-ia. The condition of having a sharp sense of smell. / oxys (keen) / osphresis / ia (a noun-forming suffix denoting a *condition*).

oss- ...   **-ossi-** ...   **osseo-** ...   Combining forms, derived from the Latin *os* (bone), genit. *ossis*, referring to *bone* or *bone tissue*.

osseo-sono-metr-y. The scientific measurement of the degree of conduction of sound through bone. / os (bone) / sonus (L. sound) / metron (G. measure) / y (a noun-forming suffix).

ossi-fication. The formation of, or conversion into, bone. / os / -ficare, facere (L. to make) / ation (a noun-forming suffix).

ossicul- ...   **ossiculo-** ...   Latin combining forms, from *ossiculum* (small bone), referring to an *ossicle, small bone of middle ear*.

ossicul-ec-tom-y. The excision of an ossicle. / ossiculum / ek (G. out) / tome (G. a cutting) / y (a noun-forming suffix indicating an *action*).

ost- ...   **oste-** ...   **osteo-** ...   Combining forms, derived from the Greek *osteon* (bone), denoting a reference to *bone* or *bone tissue*.

oste-alg-ia. Pain in a bone. / osteon (bone) / algos (G. pain) / ia (a noun-forming suffix).

ex-ost-osis. An outgrowth from the surface of a bone, consisting of bony tissue. / ex (L. out) / osteon (G. bone) / osis (G. a suffix indicating a *condition* or *disease*).

-osti- ...   **ostio-** ...   Latin combining forms, from *ostium* (opening), meaning *orifice, opening, ostium.*

inter-osti-al. Situated between openings. / inter (L. between) / ostium / al (an adjective-forming suffix).

-ot- ...   **oto-** ...   Combining forms, derived from the Greek *ous* (ear), genit. *otos*, referring to the *ear.*

peri-ot-ic. Surrounding an ear. / peri (a Greek prefix meaning *around*) / otos (ear) / ic (a Latin adjective-forming suffix).

-otic ...   An adjective-forming suffix meaning *pertaining to, affected with, causing, producing.*

hypn-otic. Inducing sleep. / hypnos (G. sleep) / otic.

-ous ...   An adjective-forming suffix, from the Latin *-osus,* meaning *characterized by, having, having a lower valence.*

poly-morph-ous. Having many forms, as a nucleus. / polys (G. many) / morphe (G. form) / ous.

-ovari- ...   **ovario-** ...   Latin combining forms, from *ovarium* (ovary), referring to the ovary.

para-ovari-an. Situated near an ovary. / para (G. near) / ovarium / an (an adjective-forming suffix indicating a *relation to something*).

ovi- ...   **ovo-** ...   Latin combining forms, from *ovum* (egg), referring to an *ovum, egg.*

ovi-par-ous. Laying eggs from which the young are hatched outside the mother's body. / ovum / parere (L. to bear) / ous (an adjective-forming suffix meaning *characterized by*).

ovul-... ovulo-... Latin combining forms, from *ovulum* (a small or young egg), meaning *ovule, young ovum.*

ovul-ation. The discharge of an ovule or young ovum from the ovary. / ovulum / ation (a Latin noun-forming suffix denoting a *process*).

-ox-... oxi-... oxid-... oxy-... Greek combining forms, from *oxys* (sharp, acid), referring to *oxygen, oxidation.*

an-ox-em-ia. A condition in which the blood lacks oxygen. / an (without) / oxys (oxygen) / haima (G. blood) / ia (a noun-forming suffix denoting a *disorder*).

oxy-... A Greek combining form, from *oxys* (sharp, pointed), meaning *pointed, sharp.*

oxy-rhine. Having a pointed nose. / oxys / rhis, genit. rhinos (G. nose).

oxy-urid. The pinworms or seatworm infesting human beings. / oxy / oura (G. tail). *Note:* in this usage, the source word *oxys* means *sharp*, in allusion to the "sharp tail" of the parasite.

oxy-... A Greek prefix, from *oxys* (keen), meaning *sharp, keen, sensitive, acute.*

oxy-aph-ia. A keen sense of touch. / oxys / haphe (G. touch) / ia (a noun-forming suffix used in names of *disorders*).

oxy-... A combining form, derived from the Greek *oxys* (acid), having reference to *acid* or to *sourness.*

oxy-gen. A colorless gas occurring in the atmosphere. / oxy / gen (a suffix meaning that which produces). *Note:* Oxygen is so called because it was formerly believed that it was essential to the formation of all acids.

oxyur-... **oxyuri-**... Greek combining forms, from *oxys* (sharp, pointed) and *oura* (tail), meaning *pinworm, thread-worm, seatworm, oxyurid.*

oxy-ur-iasis. Infestation with pinworms. / oxys / oura / iasis (a Greek suffix used to denote a *pathological condition*).

P

pachy- ...   A Greek combining form, from *pachys* (thick), meaning *thick, dense*.

pachy-derma. A thickening of the skin. / pachys / derma (G. skin).

pachy-vagin-itis. inflammation of the vagina associated with a thickening of the tissues. / pachys / vagina (L. a sheath) / itis (a suffix used to denote *inflammation*).

-palat- ...   **palati-** ...   **palato-** ...   Latin combining forms, from *palatum* (palate), referring to the *palate, roof of mouth*.

palato-gloss-al. Pertaining to the palate and the tongue. / palatum / glossa (G. tongue) / al (an adjective-forming suffix meaning *pertaining to*).

pale- ...   **paleo-** ...   Greek combining forms, from *palaios* (old), meaning *old, early, first, primitive*.

paleo-cortex. The older portion of the cortex of the brain. / palaios / cortex (L. bark, outer part).

pali- ...   **palin-** ...   Combining forms, derived from the Greek *palin* (again), meaning *backward, again*, and indicating *repetition*.

pali-lal-ia. An abnormal repetition of words or phrases. / pali (repetition) / lalein (G. speak) / ia (a noun-forming suffix).

138

palin-genesis. The appearance of an old familial characteristic in a new generation. / palin (again) / genesis (G. creation).

pall-...   palle-...   Greek combining forms, from *pallein* (to shake), referring to *vibration.*

pall-an-esthes-ia. Loss of ability to perceive vibration. / pallein / an (not, without) / aisthesis (G. perception) / ia (a noun-forming suffix used in names of *disorders*).

-palm-...   palmi-...   palmo-...   Latin combining forms, from *palma* (palm), referring to the *palm of the hand.*

palm-esthet-ic. Felt in the palm of the hand. / palma / aisthesis (G. feeling) / ic (an adjective-forming suffix meaning *characterized by*).

-palp-...   palpato-...   Latin combining forms, from *palpare* (to touch), past participle *palpatus,* meaning to *touch, feel with the hands.*

palp-able. Perceptible to the touch. / palpare / able (a suffix meaning *capable of being*).

-palpebr-...   A Latin combining form, from *palpebra* (eyelid), denoting an *eyelid.*

inter-palpebr-al. Situated between the eyelids. / inter (a Latin prefix meaning *between*) / palpebra / al (a Latin adjective forming suffix).

pan-...   pant-...   panto-...   Combining forms, derived from the Greek *pan* (genit. *pantos*), all, meaning *all, every, the whole, universal.*

pan-chromat-ic. Sensitive to light composed of all or any of the colors of the spectrum, as a photographic film. / pan (all) / chroma (G. color) / ic (an adjective forming suffix). *Note: chromat* is based on the genitive form *chromatos.*

panto-phobia. Fear of practically everything. / panto (all) /

phobos (G. fear). *Note: ia* is a noun-forming suffix denoting a condition.

pancreat- ... **pancreatico-** ... **pancreato-** ... **pancreo-** ... Greek combining forms, from *pan* (all) and *kreas*, genit. *kreatos* (flesh), referring to the *pancreas.*

pancreato-trop-ic. Having a special influence or effect on the pancreas. / pan / kreatos / tropos (G. a turning) / ic (an adjective-forming suffix meaning *characterized by*).

-papill- ... **papilli-** ... **papillo-** ... Latin combining forms, from *papilla* (small elevation), referring to a *papilla, nipple-like projection.*

papill-ec-tom-y. The surgical excision of a papilla. / papilla / ek (G. out) / tome (G. a cutting) / y (a noun-forming suffix indicating an *action*).

papul- ... **papuli-** ... **papulo-** ... Latin combining forms, from *papula* (pimple), meaning *papule, pimple.*

papuli-fer-ous. Bearing papules or pimples. / papula / ferre (bear) / ous (an adjective-forming suffix meaning *marked by*).

-par- ... **-para** ... Combining forms, derived from the Latin *parere* (bring forth), referring to *childbirth.*

par-ity. The status of a woman with regard to her having borne, or not borne, offspring. / par (give birth) / ity (a suffix denoting a *condition*).

multi-para. A woman who has borne two or more offspring in two or more pregnancies. / multi (a prefix meaning *many*) / para (childbirth).

par- ... **para-** ... Combining forms, derived from the Greek *para* (beside), meaning *adjacent to, accessory to, beyond, against, apart from, beside, abnormal, resembling.*

para-appendic-itis. Inflammation of the tissues adjacent to the appendix. / para / appendix, genit. appendicis (an appendage)

/ itis (a suffix indicating inflammation). *Note: para* in this usage means *adjacent to.*

par-onych-ia. Inflammation of the tissues beside the nail. / par (adjacent) / onyx, *genit.* onychos (a nail) / ia (a noun-forming suffix). *Note: onych* is based on the genitive form *onychos.*

-pariet- ... **parieto-** ... Latin combining forms, from *paries* (wall), genit. *parietis,* referring to the *wall of an organ or of a body cavity.*

pariet-al. Pertaining to the wall of a hollow organ or of a body cavity. / parietis / al (an adjective-forming suffix meaning *pertaining to*).

parthen- ... **partheno-** ... Greek combining forms, from *parthenos* (virgin), meaning *virgin, virginity.*

partheno-genesis. The production of offspring by virgin females, without the participation of spermatozoa. / parthenos / genesis (G. creation).

parturi- ... **parturio-** ... **parturo-** ... Combining forms, derived from the Latin *parturire* (be in labor), referring to *childbirth, labor.*

parturi-facient. A medicinal substance, or any agent, which initiates or facilitates childbirth. / parturire (be in labor) / faciens, genit. facientis (L. acting as an agent).

-patell- ... **patelli-** ... **patello-** ... Latin combining forms, from *patella* (a small pan), meaning *patella, kneecap.*

patelli-form. Shaped like a patella. / patella / forma (L. shape).

-path- ... **-pathia** ... **patho-** ... **-pathy** ... Combining forms, derived from the Greek *pathos* (disease), referring to *disease, illness, disorder.*

histo-patho-log-y. The study of small or microscopic changes in diseased tissue. / histos (G. web, tissue) / pathos (disease) /

logos (G. an account) / y (a noun-forming suffix denoting an *action* or the result of an *action*).

patri-... **patro-**...   Latin combining forms, from *pater*, genit. *patris* (father), meaning *father, male ancestor*.

patri-line-al. Descended through the male ancestors. / pater, patris / linea (L. line) / al (a Latin adjective-forming suffix).

ped-... **pedi-**... **pedo-**...   Latin combining forms, from *pes*, genit. *pedis* (foot), meaning *foot* or *footlike structure*.

pedo-path-y. Any disease of the foot. / pes, pedis / pathos (G. disease) / y (a noun-forming suffix denoting a *condition*).

-ped-... **pedo-**...   Combining forms, derived from the Greek *pais* (child), genit. *paidos*, denoting a relationship to a *child* or to *children*.

ped-iatr-ics. The branch of medicine dealing with children and children's diseases. / paidos (of a child) / iatros (G. physician) / ics (a suffix referring to a *science* or *art*).

pedicul-... **pediculi-**... **pediculo-**...   Latin combining forms, from *pediculus* (louse), referring to a *louse* or *lice*.

pedicul-osis. The condition of being infested with lice. / pediculus / osis (a Greek noun-forming suffix denoting a *condition*).

peduncul-... **pedunculi-**... **pedunculo-**...   Latin combining forms, from *pedunculus* (small foot, stalk), meaning *peduncle, stem, stalk*.

peduncul-ated. Provided with peduncles or a peduncle. / pedunculus / ated (a suffix meaning *provided with*).

pellagr-... **pellagra-**... **pellagri-**...   Combining forms, from the Latin *pellis* (skin) and the Greek *agra* (seizure), meaning *pellagra*.

pellagr-oid. A disease resembling pellagra. / pellis / agra / oeides (G. resembling).

pelv- ... **pelvi-** ... **pelvio-** ... **pelvo-** ... Latin combining forms, from *pelvis* (a basin), meaning *pelvis.*

pelvi-met-er. An instrument used for measuring the pelvis. / pelvis / metron (G. measure) / er (a suffix designating *a thing that performs a specified action*).

-pen- ... **pena-** ... **peno-** ... Latin combining forms, from *poena* (punishment), referring to *punishment, discipline, chastisement.*

philo-pen-ia. An abnormal desire to be punished. / philein (G. to love) / poena / ia (a noun-forming suffix used in names of *disorders*).

pen- ... **peni-** ... **peno-** ... Latin combining forms, from *penis* (tail), meaning *penis, phallus*

peni-schis-is. A condition in which the penis has a fissure. / penis / schisma (a split) / is (a suffix denoting a *condition*).

-penia- ... A combining form, derived from the Greek *penia* (scarcity), denoting *deficiency, dearth, poverty, scarcity.*

thrombo-penia. A deficiency of thrombin in the blood. / thrombos (G. clot) / penia (deficiency).

pent- ... **penta-** ... **penti-** ... **pento-** ... Greek combining forms, from *pente* (five), meaning *five.*

penta-valent. Having a chemical valence of five. / pente / valentia (L. strength).

-peps- ... **pept-** ... **pepto-** ... Combining forms, derived from the Greek *pepsis* (digestion) and *peptein* (to digest), referring to *digestion.*

dys-peps-ia. Impaired digestion. / dys (G. impaired) / pepsis (G. digestion) / ia (a Latin noun-forming suffix used in names of *diseases* and *disorders*).

dys-pept-ic. A person affected with dyspesia. / dys / peptein (G. to digest) / ic (a noun-forming suffix).

pepsin- ...   **pepsini-** ...   **pepsino-** ...   Greek combining forms, from *pepsis* (digestion), meaning *pepsin.*

pepsini-fer-ous. Secreting or conveying pepsin. / pepsis / ferre (L. to bear) / ous (an adjective-forming suffix meaning *characterized by*).

per- ...   A Latin prefix, from *per* (through), meaning *through, throughout, completely, excessively.*

per-colate. To cause a solvent to trickle through a medicinal substance. / per / *colatus,* past participle of *colare* (to strain).

peri- ...   A prefix of Greek origin (*peri,* around), meaning *encircling, surrounding, around.*

peri-pher-y. The outer part of something; a surrounding region. / peri (surrounding) / pherein (G. to carry) / y (a suffix forming nouns).

peri-ost-itis. Inflammation of the periosteum, the membrane surrounding a bone. / peri / osteon (G. bone) / itis (a suffix indicating inflammation).

pericard- ...   **pericardi-** ...   **pericardio-** ...   Greek combining forms, from *peri* (around, surrounding) and *kardia* (heart), referring to the *pericardium.*

pericardi-centesis. A surgical puncture of the pericardium. / peri / kardia / kentesis (G. puncture).

perine- ...   **perineo-** ...   Greek combining forms, from *perineon* (perineum), referring to the *perineum. Note: perineon* is derived from *peri* (surrounding) and *inein* (discharge, defecate).

perineo-plast-y. A plastic operation on the perineum. / perineon / plastos (G. formed) / y (a noun-forming suffix denoting an *action*).

periost-...   perioste-...   periosteo-...   Greek combining forms, from *peri* (surrounding) and *osteon* (bone), referring to the *periosteum*.

peri-oste-oma. A tumor arising from the periosteum. / peri / osteon / oma (a Greek suffix meaning *tumor*).

periton-...   peritone-...   peritoneo-...   Greek combining forms, from *peritonaion* (peritoneum), meaning *peritoneum*. *Note: peritonaion* is derived from *peri* (around) and *teinein* (to stretch).

peritoneo-centesis. The surgical puncture of the peritoneum. / peri / teinein / kentesis (G. puncture).

pero-...   A Greek combining form, from *peros* (maimed), meaning *deformed, maimed*.

pero-mania. A mania to maim and deform. / peros / mania (G. madness).

pero-cephal-us. A fetus having a deformed head. / peros / kephale (G. head) / us (a Latin noun ending meaning *one who*).

-petal...   A Latin suffix, from *petere* (to seek) and *al* (an adjective-forming suffix), meaning *moving toward, seeking*.

cortico-petal. Moving toward the cortex. / cortex, corticis (L. a cortex) / petere / al.

petr-...   petro-...   petros-...   Latin combining forms, from *petra* (stone) and *petrosus* (stony), referring to the *petrous portion of the temporal bone.*

petr-ous. Hard as a stone; rocky. / petra / ous (an adjective-forming suffix meaning *having the characteristics of*).

petros-ec-tom-y. Excision of a part of the petrous portion of the temporal bone. / petrosus / ek (G. out) / tome (G. a cutting) / y (a noun-forming suffix denoting an *action*).

petri- . . .   **petro-** . . .   Latin combining forms, from *petra* (rock), meaning *hard, rocky.*

petri-faction. Conversion to a hard or stony substance. / petra / factio (L. a making).

-pexia . . .   **-pexis** . . .   Greek combining forms, from *pexis* (a fixation), meaning *fixation, attachment, securing.*

nephro-pexy. Fixation or attachment of a loose kidney. / nephros (G. kidney) / pexis (fixation).

-phac- . . .   **phaco-** . . .   Greek combining forms, from *phakos* (a lentil), referring to a *lens,* especially the *crystalline lens of the eye.*

phaco-cele. A herniation of the crystalline lens. / phakos / kele (G. hernia, swelling). *Note:* the allusion to "lentil" is based on the resemblance, with regard to shape, between a typical convex lens and a lentil.

-phag- . . .   **-phagia** . . .   **phago-** . . .   **-phagy** . . .   Combining forms, derived from the Greek *phagein* (to eat), referring to *eating, ingestion, engulfing.*

mono-phag-ism. Subsistence on, or the eating of, one kind of food. / monos (G. single) / phagein (eat) / ism (a Latin noun-forming suffix denoting a *condition, process*).

-phalang- . . .   **phalange-** . . .   **phalangi-** . . .   **phalango-** . . . Greek combining forms from *phalanx,* genit. *phalangos* (line of battle, log), referring to the bones or a *bone of a finger or a toe.*

sym-phalang-ism. An abnormal fusion of the bones of a finger or a toe. / sym, syn (a Greek prefix meaning *together with*) / phalangos / ism (a noun-forming suffix designating a *condition*).

-phall-... phalli-... phallo-... Greek combining forms, from *phallos* (penis), meaning *phallus, penis.*

phall-ic-ism. The worship of the phallus as a symbol of generative power. / phallos / ic (an adjective-forming suffix meaning *pertaining to*) / ism (a noun-forming suffix denoting an *act*).

phaner-... phanero-... Greek combining forms, from *phaneros* (visible), meaning *visible, manifest, open, apparent.*

phanero-phil-ia. Fondness for bodily exposure. / phaneros / philein (G. to love) / ia (a noun-forming suffix denoting a *state, condition*).

pharmac-... pharmaceutic-... pharmaco-... Combining forms, derived from the Greek *pharmakon* (drug) and pharmakeutikos (pertaining to drugs), relating to *drugs, medicinal substances.*

pharmaco-dynam-ics. The study of the action of drugs. / pharmakon (drug) / dynamis (G. power) / ics (a noun-forming plural suffix, also used in the singular, indicating a *study*).

-pharyng-... pharynge-... pharyngo-... Greek combining forms, from *pharynx*, genit. *pharyngos* (pharynx, throat), meaning *pharynx, throat.*

pharyng-ismus. A spasm of the muscles of the pharynx. / pharyngos / ismus (L. a suffix used to denote an *abnormal condition, as a spasm*).

-phasia... A Greek terminal combining form, from *phasis* (speech), meaning *speech, utterance.*

brady-phas-ia. Abnormal slowness of speech. / bradys (G. slow) / phasis / ia (a noun-forming suffix denoting a *disorder*).

phenol-...   phenolo-...   Greek combining forms, from *phainein* (to shine), meaning *phenol, carbolic acid.*

phen-ol-phtha-l-ein. A substance used as an indicator, laxative, etc. / phainein / ol (a chemical suffix used to denote an alcohol or phenol) / naphtha (G. a petroleum distillate) / al (a chemical suffix denoting an aldehyde, alcohol, etc.) / ein (a variant of *in,* designating several groups of chemical substances). *Note:* the combining form *phen* (from *phainein,* to shine) was first used to denote derivation from coal tar, a byproduct in the production of illuminating gas, in allusion to the "shining" quality of the flame produced by the gas.

-phil-...   phila-...   -phile...   -philia...   philo-...
-philous...   -philus...   -phily...   Greek combining forms, from *philein* (to love) and *philos* (loving), meaning *loving, liking, preferring, having an affinity for, one who loves.*

andro-phil-ous. Preferring men; having a predilection for men. / aner, genit. andros (male) / philein / ous (adjective-forming suffix meaning *having*).

phleb-...   phlebo-...   Greek combining forms, from *phleps* (vein), genit. *phlebos,* meaning *vein, venous.*

phlebo-stasis. A stagnation of blood in a vein. / phlebos / stasis (G. a standing).

phlog-...   phlogo-...   Greek combining forms, from *phlox,* genit. phlogos (fire), meaning *inflammation.*

phlog-istic. Marked by inflammation. / phlox, phlogos / istic (an adjective-forming suffix meaning *characterized by*).

phlycten-...   phlycteno-...   Combining forms, derived from the Greek *phlyktaina* (a blister), denoting a reference to a *blister, vesicle* or *pustule.*

phlycten-oid. Resembling a blister or vesicle. / phlyktaina (blister) / oides (L. likeness in form).

phlycten-ule. A small blister. / phlyktaina / ulus (a noun-forming suffix indicating *dimunitive size*).

-phobia . . .   phobo- . . .   Greek combining forms, from *phobos* (fear), referring to *fear, aversion for.*

patho-phob-ia. Abnormal fear of illness. / pathos (G. disease) / phobos / ia (a Latin noun-forming suffix used in names of *disorders*).

phon- . . .   -phonc . . .   phono- . . .   -phony . . .   Greek combining forms, from *phone* (sound), referring to *sound, voice sound.*

osteo-phone. A type of hearing aid utilizing bone conduction. / osteon (G. bone) / phone (a device for transmitting sound).

-phor- . . .   -phora . . .   -phore . . .   -phoresis . . .   -phoria . . . **phoro- . . .   -phorous . . .   -phorus . . .**   Combining forms, derived from the Greek *pherein* (to bear), indicating *motion, direction, a bearer, bearing.*

eu-phor-ous. Having a feeling of euphoria or well-being. / eu (a prefix meaning *well*) / pherein (to bear) / ous (an adjective-forming suffix).

phos-phor-ous. Exhibiting phosphorescence. / phos (G. light) / pherein / ous (an adjective-forming suffix).

phos- . . .   photo- . . .   Greek combining forms, from *phos*, genit. *photos* (light), meaning *light*.

photo-phob-ia. Abnormal sensitivity to light, said especially of the eye. / phos, photos / phobos (G. fear) / ia (a noun-forming suffix used in names of *disorders*).

-phosph- . . .   phosphat- . . .   phospho- . . .   phosphor- . . . **phosphoro- . . .**   Greek combining forms, from *phos* (light) and *pherein* (to bear), referring to *phosphorus, phosphoric acid, phosphate.*

phosph-at-em-ia. A condition marked by an increase in the amount of phosphates in the blood. / phos / pherein / ate (a chemical suffix denoting a salt of phosphoric acid, i.e., a phosphate) / haima (G. blood) / ia (a noun-forming suffix used in names of *disorders*).

-phren-... phrenic-... phrenico-... phreno-... Combining forms, derived from the Greek *phren*, genit. *phrenos* (mind, diaphragm), referring to the *diaphragm*, the *mind. Note:* the diaphragm was thought to be the seat of the intellect.

sub-phren-ic. Situated under the diaphragm. / sub (a Latin prefix meaning *beneath*) / phren (diaphragm) / ic (a Latin adjective-forming suffix).

schizo-phren-ia. A type of psychotic disorder; dementia precox. / schizein (G. to split) / phren (mind) / ia (a Latin noun-forming suffix used in names of *diseases* and *disorders*).

phthir-... A Greek combining form, from *phtheir* (louse), meaning *louse, lice.*

phthir-iasis. The condition of being infested with lice. / phtheir / iasis (Greek suffix denoting a *condition,* usually *pathologic*).

phthisic-... phthisio-... Greek combining forms, from *phthisikos* (affected with tuberculosis), referring to *wasting, tuberculosis.*

phthisio-phob-ia. Abnormal fear of tuberculosis. / phthisikos / phobos (G. fear) / ia (a noun-forming suffix denoting a *disorder*).

-phyl-... phylo-... Greek combining forms, from *phylon* (race), referring to a *tribe, clan, phylum.*

phylo-geny. The history of the development of a race. / phylon

/ geny (a suffix meaning *development of*, from the Greek *gignes-thai*, to become).

-phylact- ... **phylacto-** ... Greek combining forms, from *phylassein* (to defend) and *phylaktikos* (guarding), referring to *protection, defense, preservation*.

pro-phylact-ic. A medicine, or any agent, which prevents or guards against a disease. / pro (before) / phylaktikos / ic (a noun-forming suffix).

-phyll- ... **phyllo-** ... Greek combining forms, from *phyllon* (leaf), referring to a *leaf* or to a *leaflike structure*.

chloro-phyll. The green pigment of leaves. / chloros (G. green) / phyllon.

phys- ... **physic-** ... **physico-** ... **physio-** ... Greek combining forms, from *physis* (nature), referring to *nature, physical agents, facial expression*.

physio-gnom-y. Facial features and expression, especially as a sign of character. / physis / gnomon (G. one who knows) / y (a suffix denoting a *condition, quality*).

-phyt- ... **-phyte** ... **phyto-** ... Greek combining forms, from *phyton* (plant), meaning *plant, vegetable*.

tricho-phyt-osis. Infection with the ringworm fungus. / thrix, genit. trichos (G. hair) / phyton / osis (a noun-forming suffix denoting a *disorder*).

picr- ... **picro-** ... Combining forms, derived from the Greek *pikros* (bitter), meaning *bitter*.

picro-geus-ia. An abnormal sensation of a bitter taste. / pikros (G. bitter) / geusis (G. taste) / ia (a noun-forming suffix used to indicate a disorder).

pict- ... **picto-** ...   Latin combining forms, from *pingere,* past participle *pictus* (to paint), meaning *paint, picture, depict.*

picto-therapy. The use of painting as a means of therapy. / pictus / therapeia (G. therapy).

-pies- ... **piesi-** ... **pieso-** ... **piez-** ... **piezo-** ...   Greek combining forms, from *piezein* (to press) and *piesis* (pressure), meaning *pressure.*

pies-esthes-ia. The perception of pressure. / piesis / aisthesis (G. feeling, perception) / ia (a noun-forming suffix denoting a *condition*).

-pil- ... **pilo-** ...   Latin combining forms, from *pilus* (hair), meaning *hair.*

de-pil-atory. A substance which removes hair. / de (a prefix meaning *off*) / pilus / atory (a noun-forming suffix designating an agent which does a specified *activity*).

-pimel- ... **pimelo-** ...   Greek combining forms, from *pimele* (fat), referring to *fat, fatness, fatty tissue.*

pimel-oma. A tumor composed of fat or fatty tissue. / pimele / oma (G. tumor, swelling).

pinn- ... **pinnati-** ...   Latin combining forms, from *pinna* (feather), meaning *fin, feather.*

pinn-ate. Of a plant, having leaflets in a featherlike arrangement. / pinna / ate (an adjective-forming suffix meaning *shaped like*).

pisci- ...   A Latin combining form, from *piscis* (fish), meaning *fish.*

pisci-vor-ous. Eating mainly fish. / piscis / vorare (L. to eat) / ous (an adjective-forming suffix meaning *characterized by*).

pituit- ... **pituitari-** ... **pituito-** ... **pituitr-** ...   Latin combining forms, from *pituita* (phlegm, mucus) and *pituitari-*

us (pertaining to mucus), referring to the *pituitary gland, hypophysis.*

pituitar-ism. A condition resulting from an excessive activity of the pituitary gland. / pituitarius / ism (a Latin or Greek suffix denoting an *abnormal condition*).

-placent-... **placenti-**... **placento-**... Latin combining forms, from *placenta* (a cake), meaning *placenta* (in allusion to its shape, which resembles that of a flat cake).

placent-ation. The development and attachment of the placenta. / placenta / ation (a noun-forming suffix denoting an *act* or *process*).

-plasia... **-plasis**... Combining forms, derived from the Greek *plassein* (to mold) and *plasis* (a molding), referring to *development, change, growth.*

hypo-plasia. Deficient growth or development. / hypo (G. deficiency) / plassein (to mold).

-plasm-... **plasma-**... **plasmo-**... Greek combining forms, from *plasma* (a formed substance), referring to *plasma, protoplasm.*

proto-plasm-ic. Pertaining to protoplasm. / protos (G. first) / plasma / ic (an adjective-forming suffix meaning *pertaining to*).

-plasty... A Greek terminal combining form, from *plassein* (to form, mold) and *plastos* (formed), referring to *plastic surgery, repair, formation.*

blepharo-plasty. A plastic operation on an eyelid. / blepharon (G. eyelid) / plastos.

platy-... A Greek prefix, from *platys* (broad), meaning *wide, broad, flat.*

platy-cephal-ic. Having a wide head. / platys / kephale (G. head) / ic (an adjective-forming suffix meaning *characterized by*).

-plegia ...   A Greek combining form, from *plege* (a stroke), meaning *paralysis, stroke, blow*.

quadri-pleg-ia. Paralysis of all four limbs. / quattuor (L. four) / plege / ia (a Latin noun-forming suffix used in names of *diseases*).

pleio- ...   **pleo-** ...   Greek combining forms, from *pleion* (more), meaning *more, increased, excess*.

pleo-cyt-osis. An increase in the number of cells. / pleion / kytos (G. cell) / osis (a noun-forming suffix denoting a *disorder*).

-pleur- ...   **pleura-** ...   **pleuro-** ...   Greek combining forms, from *pleura* (rib, side), meaning *pleura*.

pleuro-centesis. A surgical puncture of the pleura. / pleura / kentesis (G. puncture).

-plic- ...   **plica-** ...   **plici-** ...   **plicato-** ...   Latin combining forms, from *plicare*, past participle *plicatus* (to fold), meaning *ridge, fold*.

du-plic-ation. A folding in two. / duo (L. two) / plicare / ation (a Latin noun-forming suffix denoting an *action* or *process*).

-ploid ...   A suffix, derived from the Greek *ploos* (-fold) and *eidos* (form, shape), referring to a *multiple of chromosomes*.

di-ploid. Having twice the number of chromosomes normally occurring in a mature reproductive cell. / di (G. twice) / ploos (-fold) / eidos (G. form).

plumb- ...   **plumbi-** ...   Latin combining forms, from *plumbum* (lead), meaning *lead*.

plumbi-ferous. Bearing or containing lead. / plumbum / ferre (L. to bear) / ous (an adjective-forming suffix denoting a *characteristic*).

pluri- ...   A Latin prefix, from *plus* (more), genit. *pluris*, meaning *several, many, more*.

pluri-nucle-ar. Having several nuclei. / pluris / nuculeus (L. diminutive of *nux* (nut), genit. *nucis*) / ar (an adjective-forming suffix meaning *relating to*).

pluto-... A Greek combining form, from *ploutos* (wealth), meaning *wealth, riches*.

pluto-mania. An unfounded belief that one is very wealthy. / ploutos / mania (G. madness).

-pnea... pneo-... Combining forms, derived from the Greek *pnein* (to breathe), indicating a reference to *breathing, respiration*.

dys-pnea. Difficult breathing; shortness of breath. / dys (a Greek prefix denoting *difficulty*) / pnein (to breathe).

pneum-... pneuma-... pneumato-... pneumo-... Combining forms, based on the Greek *pneuma* (genit. *pneumatos*), air, referring to *respiration, air, gas*.

pneum-arthr-osis. A condition marked by the presence of air, or any gas, within the cavity of a joint. / pneum (air) / arthron (G. joint) / osis (a Greek suffix denoting a *condition or disorder*).

pneumato-cele. A sac, swelling, or any mass containing air (or any gas). / pneumato (of gas) / kele (G. swelling, rupture).

pneumo-graph. An apparatus for recording respiratory movements. / pneumo (respiration) / graphein (G. to write, record).

pneumo-... pneumon-... pneumono-... Greek combining forms, from *pneumon* (lung), meaning *lung*.

pneumo-coni-osis. A disease of the lung caused by inhalation of dust. / pneumon / konia (G. dust) / osis (a Greek suffix forming nouns denoting an abnormal *condition*).

-pod-... podi-... podo-... -podium... -podous... Greek combining forms, from *pous*, genit. *podos* (foot), referring to the *foot* or a *footlike structure*.

podo-gram. A print or outline of the foot. / pous, podos / gramma (G. letter, something recorded).

-poiesis ... poietic ... Greek combining forms, from *poiesis* (a making), referring to *production, formation, making.*

chole-poiesis. Formation of bile. / chole (G. bile) / poiesis.

poikilo- ... A Greek combining form, from *poikilos* (varied), meaning *irregular, varied in shape.*

poikilo-cyte. A red blood cell having an irregular shape. / poikilos / kytos (G. vessel, cell).

polio- ... A Greek combining form, from *polios* (gray), referring to the *gray matter of the nervous system.*

polio-en-cephalo-path-y. Any disease of the gray matter of the brain. / polios / en (in) / kephale (G. head) / pathos (G. disease) / y (a noun-forming suffix denoting a *condition*).

pollic- ... pollici- ... Latin combining forms, from *pollex* (thumb), genit. *pollicis,* referring to the *thumb.*

pollici-form. Having the shape of a thumb. / pollicis / forma (L. form, shape).

pollin- ... pollini- ... Latin combining forms, from *pollen,* genit. *pollinis* (pollen), meaning *pollen.*

pollini-fer-ous. Bearing pollen. / pollinis / ferre (L. bear) / ous (an adjective-forming suffix designating a *characteristic*).

poly- ... A Greek prefix, from *polys* (many), meaning *much, many, several, excessive.*

poly-morpho-nucle-ar. Having nuclei of several forms. / polys / morphos (G. form) / nucleus (L. kernel, nucleus) / ar (an adjective-forming suffix meaning *of the nature of*).

pono- ... A Greek combining form, from *ponos* (toil), referring to *work, toil, exertion.*

pono-metr-y. Measurement of exertion. / ponos / metron (G. measure) / y (a noun-forming suffix denoting an *action*).

-pont- ...   **ponto-** ...   Latin combining forms, from *pons,* genit. *pontis* (a bridge), referring to the *pons.*

sub-pont-ine. Situated below the pons. / sub (L. beneath) / pontis / ine (a suffix used to form adjectives).

porne- ...   **porno-** ...   Greek combining forms, from *porne* (harlot), meaning *prostitute, whore, harlot.*

porno-graph-y. Writings, or other visual materials, intended mainly to arouse sexual desire or to provide sexual titillation. / porne / graphein (G. to write) / y (a noun-forming suffix denoting an *action*).

post- ...   A prefix, derived from the Latin *post* (after), meaning *later, behind, following, after.*

post-nasal. Situated or occurring behind (or in the back of) the nose. / post / nasus (L. nose) / al (an adjective-forming suffix).

post-partum. Occurring after or following childbirth. / post / parturire (L. be in labor).

postero- ...   A Latin prefix, from *posterus* (behind), meaning *behind, in the back, posterior,*

postero-lateral. In the back and to the side. / posterus / lateralis (L. to the side).

pre- ...   A combining form, derived from the Latin *prae* (before), meaning *in front, anterior, earlier, prior, before.*

pre-cordi-al. Pertaining to the region of the chest in front of the heart. / pre (in front) / cor, *genit.* cordis (L. the heart) / al (an adjective-forming suffix).

pre-medic-al. Given or taken before the regular medical courses. / pre (prior) / medicare (L. to heal) / al (an adjective-forming suffix).

presby- ...   A Greek combining form, from *presbys* (old), meaning *old, old age.*

presby-op-ia. The impairment of vision characteristic of old age. / presbys / ops (G. eye) / ia (a noun-forming suffix used in names of *disorders*).

presso- ...   **pressur-** ...   **pressuro-** ...   Latin combining forms, from *pressura* (pressure), referring to *pressure.*

presso-meter. An instrument used to measure pressure. / pressura / metron (G. measure) / er (a suffix denoting *a thing that performs a specified function*).

primi- ...   A Latin combining form, from *primus* (first), meaning *first time.*

primi-para. A woman who is giving birth for the first time. / primus / parere (L. to bear).

prism- ...   **prismat-** ...   **prismato-** ...   Latin combining forms, from *prisma,* genit. *prismatos* (prism), meaning *prism, prismatic lens.*

prismato-met-er. An instrument for measuring prisms. / prismatos / metron (G. measure) / er (person or *thing performing a specified action*).

pro- ...   A preflx, derived from the Greek pro (before), meaning *in front of, occurring before, before.*

pro-cephal-ic. Pertaining to the front part of the head; in front of the head. / pro (in front of) / kephale (G. head) / ic (an adjective-forming suffix).

pro-drome. A premonitory sign or symptom, as of a disease. / pro (before) / dromos (G. running).

proct- ...   **procto-** ...   Greek combining forms, from *proktos* (anus), meaning *rectum, anus.*

proct-ectas-ia. An abnormal dilatation of the rectum. / proktos / ektasis (G. dilatation, extension) / ia (a noun-forming suffix used in names of *disorders*).

prosop-...   **prosopo-...**   Greek combining forms, from *prosopon* (face), meaning *face, countenance.*

prosop-a-gnos-ia. Inability to recognize faces. / prosopon / a (not) / gnosis (G. knowledge) / ia (a Latin noun-forming suffix denoting a *disorder*).

prostat-...   **prostatico-...**   **prostato-...**   Greek combining forms, from *prostates* (one or something standing before), *pro* (before) and *histanai* (stand), referring to the *prostate gland.*

prostat-ec-tom-y. Surgical excision of the prostate. / prostates / ek (G. out) / tome (G. a cutting) / y (a noun-forming suffix denoting an *action*).

prosth-...   **prosthet-...**   **prostho-...**   Greek combining forms, from *prosthesis* (an addition) and *prosthetos* (put on), referring to an *artificial body structure, prosthesis.*

prosth-odont-ics. Branch of dentistry dealing with artificial teeth, crowns, etc. / prosthesis / odous, genit. odontos (a tooth) / ics (a suffix denoting a specified *science*).

prot-...   **proto-...**   Combining forms, derived from the Greek *protos* (first), meaning *earliest, original, primitive, first.*

proto-plasm. The viscid material forming the essential substance of living cells. / protos (first) / plasma (G. something formative).

protein-...   **proteino-...**   **proteo-...**   Greek combining forms, from *proteios* (prime, chief) and *in* (a chemical suffix), meaning *protein.*

protein-ase. An enzyme aiding in the digestion of proteins. / proteios / in / ase (a noun-forming suffix denoting an *enzyme*).

proxim- ...   **proximo-** ...   Latin combining forms, from *proximus* (next), meaning *nearest, closest, next.*

proxim-ad. Directed toward a proximal part or a center. / proximus / ad (to, toward).

prurit- ...   **prurito-** ...   Latin combining forms, from *prurire* (to itch), past participle *pruritus*, referring to an *itch* or *itching.*

prurit-ic. Marked by itching. / pruritus / ic (a Latin adjective-forming suffix meaning *characterized by*).

pseud- ...   **pseudo-** ...   Greek combining forms, from *pseudein* (deceive), meaning *false, deceptive, illusory, spurious.*

pseudo-edema. A puffiness resembling edema. / pseudein / oidema (G. swelling).

psych- ...   **-psycho-** ...   Greek combining forms, from *psyche* (mind, soul), meaning *mind, psyche, mental condition.*

psych-a-sthen-ia. A type of neurosis marked by lack of self-control. / psyche / a (without) / sthenos (G. strength) / ia (a noun-forming suffix used in names of diseases).

psychro- ...   A combining form, derived from the Greek *psychros* (cold), referring to *cold, low temperature.*

psychro-esthes-ia. A condition in which a part of the body feels or seems to be cold although it is warm. / psychros (cold) / aisthesis (G. feeling, sensation) / ia (a Latin noun-forming suffix used in names of *diseases* and *disorders*).

pterig- ...   **pterigo-** ...   Greek combining forms, from *pteryx* (a wing), genit. *pterygos*, referring to a *wing, winglike structure, pterygoid process.*

pteryg-oid. Shaped like a wing. / pterygos / eides (G. having form of).

-ptern- ...   **pterno-** ...   Greek combining forms, from *pterna* (heel), referring to the *heel.*

pterno-helc-osis. Ulceration of the heel. / pterna / helkos (G. ulcer) / osis (a Greek noun-forming suffix denoting a *condition, disorder*).

ptoch- ...   **ptochi-** ...   **ptocho-** ...   Greek combining forms, from *ptochos* (a beggar), meaning *poor, poverty.*

ptocho-phil-ous. Afflicting mainly the poor. / ptochos / philein (G. to love) / ous (an adjective-forming suffix meaning *characterized by*).

-ptosis ...   A combining form, derived from the Greek *ptosis* (a falling), denoting a *downward displacement, drooping, sagging.*

viscero-ptosis. An abnormal downward displacement of the abdominal organs. / viscus, pl. viscera (L. internal organ) / ptosis (downward displacement).

-ptyal- ...   **ptyalo-** ...   Greek combining forms, from *ptyalon* (spittle), referring to *saliva.*

ptyal-agogue. A substance which stimulates the formation of saliva. / ptyalon / agogue (something that incites or stimulates, from *agein*, to lead).

pub- ...   **pubio-** ...   **pubo-** ...   Latin combining forms, from *pubes* (hair on the genital organs, hence, by extension, the region of the genitals), referring to the *pubic bones, pubic hair.*

pubio-tom-y. The surgical cutting of the symphysis pubis, the juncture between the two pubic bones. / pubes / tome (G. a cutting) / y (a noun-forming suffix denoting an *action*).

puber- ...   **pubert-** ...   **puberto-** ...   Latin combining forms, from *pubertas* (adulthood), meaning *puberty*

puberto-trich-ia. The growth of hair characteristic of puberty. / pubertas / thrix, genit. trichos (G. hair) / ia (a noun-forming suffix used in names of *conditions*).

pudend- . . .   **pudendi-** . . .   **pudendo-** . . .   Latin combining forms, from *pudendus* (something to be ashamed of), referring to the *pudendum, genital organs of the female.*

pudend-alg-ia. Pain in the genital organs of the female. / pudendus / algos (G. pain) / ia (a Latin noun-forming suffix used in names of *disorders*).

puerper- . . .   A combining form, derived from the Latin *puerpera* (woman in childbirth), referring to *childbirth* or the *period following childbirth.*

puer-per-al-ism. Any disorder resulting from childbirth. / puer (L. child) / parere (L. to bear) / al (a Latin adjective-forming suffix) / ism (a noun-forming suffix, from the Latin, denoting a *condition*).

pul- . . .   **pulic-** . . .   **pulici-** . . .   Latin combining forms, from *pulex*, genit. *pulicis* (a flea), meaning *flea.*

de-pul-ization. The process of freeing from fleas. / de (away) / pulex / ization (a noun-forming suffix denoting a *process*).

pulmo- . . .   **pulmon-** . . .   **pulmono-** . . .   Latin combining forms, from *pulmo*, genit. *pulmonis* (lung), meaning *lung.*

pulmon-ec-tom-y. Excision of a lung. / pulmonis / ek (G. out) / tome (G. a cutting) / y (a noun-forming suffix denoting an *action*).

pulp- . . .   **pulpi-** . . .   **pulpo-** . . .   Latin combining forms, from *pulpa* (flesh), referring to *dental pulp.*

pulp-alg-ia. Pain in the pulp of a tooth. / pulpa / algos (pain) / ia (a noun-forming suffix used in names of *disorders*).

punct- . . .   **puncti-** . . .   **puncto-** . . .   Latin combining forms, from *punctum* (point), referring to a *point, dot.*

puncti-form. Resembling a point or dot. / punctum / forma (L. shape, form).

-pupill-... pupillo-... Latin combining forms, from *pupilla* (pupil), referring to the *pupil of the eye.*

pupill-a-ton-ia. A condition in which the pupil does not react to light. / pupilla / a (without) / tonos (G. tension) / ia (a noun-forming suffix used in names of *disorders*).

-pur-... puri-... Latin combining forms, from *pus*, genit. *puris* (pus), meaning *pus.*

pur-ulent. Containing pus. / pus, puris / ulent (a Latin suffix, from *ulentus,* meaning *full of*).

pustul-... pustuli-... pustulo-... Latin combining forms, from *pustula* (pustule), meaning *pustule.*

pustul-ant. A substance which causes the formation of pustules. / pustula / ant (a Latin noun-forming suffix meaning *a thing that does*).

-py-... pyo-... Greek combining forms, from *pyon* (pus), meaning *pus.*

py-ur-ia. The presence of pus in the urine. / pyon / ouron (G. urine) / ia (a noun-forming suffix used in names of *diseases*).

pyel-... pyelo-... Greek combining forms, from *pyelos* (basin), referring to the *pelvis of the kidney.*

pyel-ectasis. An abnormal dilatation of the pelvis of the kidney. / pyelos / ektasis (G. distention).

-pyg-... pygo-... Combining forms, derived from the Greek *pyge* (rump), referring to the *buttocks.*

steato-pyg-ia. The condition of having excessive fat on the buttocks. / stear, genit. steatos (G. fat) / pyge (rump) / ia (a noun-forming suffix used in *names of disorders*).

pykn-... pykno-... Greek combining forms, from *pyknos* (thick), meaning *thick, compact, solid, frequent.*

pykn-osis. The shrinking and thickening of a nucleus of a cell. / pyknos / osis (a suffix denoting an abnormal condition).

-pyl-...   pyle-...   pylo-...   pylephleb-...   Greek combining forms, from *pyle* (gate) and *phleps*, genit. *phlebos* (vein), referring to the *portal vein.*

pyle-phleb-ectasis. An abnormal dilatation of the portal vein. / pyle / phlebos / ektasis (G. dilatation).

-pylor-...   pyloro-...   Greek combining forms, from pyloros (gatekeeper), referring to the *pylorus.*

pyloro-spasm. A spastic contraction of the pylorus. / pyloros / spasmos (G. a spasm).

...   Greek combining forms, from *pyretos* (fever), referring to *fever, heat.*

pyreto-gen. A substance which produces fever. / pyretos / gen (G. that which produces).

-pyr-...   pyre-...   pyret-...   pyreto-...   pyrex-...   pyro--pyth-...   pytho-...   Combining forms, derived from the Greek *pythein* (to rot), denoting a reference to *decomposition, decay, rot.*

pytho-phil-ic. Thriving in filth or decaying matter. / pythein (rot) / philein (G. to love) / ic (a Latin adjective-forming suffix).

Q

quadr- ... **quadri-** ... Latin combining forms, from *quattuor* (four), meaning *four*.

quadri-ceps. Having four heads, as a muscle. / quattuor / caput (L. head).

quadrant- ... **quadranto-** ... Latin combining forms, from *quadrans*, genit. *quadrantis* (quarter), meaning *quarter, one fourth*.

quadrant-an-op-ia. Defective vision in one fourth of the visual field. / quadrantis / an (without) / ops (G. eye) / ia (a noun-forming suffix used in names of *disorders*).

quinque- ... A Latin combining form, from *quinque* (five), meaning *five*.

quinque-cuspid. A tooth having five cusps. / quinque / cuspis (L. a point).

quint- ... **quinti-** ... **quintu-** ... Latin combining forms, from *quintus* (fifth), meaning *fifth*.

quinti-gravida. A woman who is pregnant for the fifth time. / quintus / gravida (L. heavy with child).

R

rab- ... **rabi-** ... Latin combining forms, from *rabies* (madness), meaning *rabies*.

rabi-phylact-ic. Preventing rabies. / rabies / phylakterion (G. safeguard) / ic (an adjective-forming suffix meaning *producing*).

rachi- ... **rachio-** ... Greek combining forms, from *rachis* (spine), referring to the *spine, spinal column*.

rachio-campsis. Curvature of the spine. / rachis / kampsis (G. a bending).

radi- ... **radio-** ... Latin combining forms, from *radius* (a rod), referring to a *radius* or the *radius of the forearm*.

radi-al. Pertaining to the radius. / radius / al (a Latin adjective-forming suffix meaning *pertaining to*).

radici- ... **radico-** ... **radicul-** ... **radiculo-** ... Latin combining forms, from *radix*, genit. *radicis* (a root), meaning *root, rootlike structure*.

radico-tom-y. The surgical cutting of a root. / radicis / tome (G. a cutting) / y (a noun-forming suffix indicating an *action*).

radio- ... A Latin combining form, from *radius* (ray), referring to *radiation, radiant energy, radium*.

radio-act-ive. Capable of giving off radiant energy. / radius / agere (L. to do), past participle *actus* / ive (an adjective-forming suffix meaning *having the quality of*).

ram- ...   **rami-** ...   Combining forms, derived from the Latin *ramus* (a branch), designating an involvement of a *branch* or *root*.

ram-itis. Inflammation of a root, as of a nerve. / ramus (root) / itis (a suffix denoting *inflammation*).

rami-section. The surgical cutting of a root or branch. / ramus / secare (L. to cut), past participle *sectus* / ion (a noun-forming suffix denoting an *action*).

re- ...   A prefix of Latin origin, meaning *back, backwards, again, anew*.

re-tract. To draw back. / re (back) / tractare (L. to draw).

re-pell-ent. A substance which drives something back. / re / pellere (L. to drive) / ent (a noun-forming suffix).

-rect- ...   **recto-** ...   Latin combining forms, from *rectum* (straight), meaning *rectum*.

recto-cele. A hernia of the rectum. / rectum / kele (G. hernia).

-reflex- ...   **reflexi-** ...   **reflexo-** ...   Latin combining forms, from *reflectere*, past participle *reflexus* (to reflect), meaning *reflex, reflex action*.

a-reflex-ia. A condition in which reflexes are absent. / a (without) / re (back) / flectere (L. to bend) / ia (a noun-forming suffix used in names of *disorders*).

refract- ...   **refracto-** ...   **refrang-** ...   Latin combining forms, from *refringere*, past participle *refractus* (to turn aside), meaning *refraction*.

re-frang-ible. That can be refracted; amenable to refraction. / re (back) / frangere (L. to break) / ible (a Latin suffix having the same meaning as *able*).

ren- . . .   **reni-** . . .   **reno-** . . .   Latin combining forms, from *ren* (kidney), meaning *kidney.*

reni-puncture. The surgical puncture of the capsule of the kidney. / ren / punctura (L. a pricking).

respir- . . .   **respirat-** . . .   **respiro-** . . .   Latin combining forms, from *respirare,* past participle *respiratus* (to breathe), referring to *respiration, breathing.*

respiro-met-er. An instrument used to measure respiratory movements. / respirare / metron (G. measure) / er (a suffix meaning *something that does*).

ret- . . .   **reti-** . . .   Latin combining forms, from *rete* (a net), plural *retia,* referring to a *netlike structure, network, rete.*

reti-ation. The formation of a network. / retia / ation (a Latin noun-forming suffix denoting an *action*)

reticul- . . .   **reticulo-** . . .   Latin combining forms, from *reticulum* (a small net), referring to a *network, net, reticulum.*

reticulo-cyte. A young red blood cell having a filamentous network. / reticulum / kytos (G. cell).

reticulocyt- . . .   **reticulocyto-** . . .   Combining forms, from the Latin *reticulum* (a small net) and the Greek *kytos* (a cell), referring to a young red blood cell showing a filamentous network, i.e. a *reticulocyte.*

reticulo-cyto-pen-ia. An abnormal decrease in the number of reticulocytes. / reticulum / kytos / penia (G. poverty) / ia (a noun-forming suffix denoting a *condition*)

retin- . . .   **retino-** . . .   Latin combining forms, from *rete,* genitive *retis* (a net), meaning *retina.*

ret-ina. The innermost layer of the wall of the eyeball. / retis / ina (a suffix used in forming *feminine nouns*).

retino-path-y. Any disease of the retina. / retis / ina / pathos (G. disease) / y (a noun-forming suffix denoting a *condition*).

retro- . . . A prefix, derived from the Latin *retro* (back, backward), meaning *back, backward, behind.*

retro-grade. Recede; move backward. / retro (backward) / gradi (L. to walk).

retro-auricul-ar. Situated behind an auricle. / retro / auricula (L. a small ear).

rhabd- . . . **rhabdo-** . . . Greek combining forms, from *rhabdos* (a rod), referring to a *striated muscle fiber, rodlike structure.*

rhabdo-my-oma. A tumor derived from striated muscle fibers. / rhabdos / mys (G. muscle) / oma (G. a tumor).

rheo- . . . A Greek combining form, from *rheos* (current), meaning *current, electric current, flow.*

rheo-stat. An instrument for controlling the strength of an electric current. / rheos / states (G. causing to stand).

rheumat- . . . **rheumato-** . . . Greek combining forms, from *rheuma,* genitive *rheumatos* (a discharge, a flowing of body "humours"), referring to *rheumatism.*

rheumat-ism. A popular term for a variety of disorders marked by painful and swollen joints. / rheumatos / ismos (G. an abnormal condition).

rheumat-oid. Resembling rheumatism. / rheumatos / eides (G. having the form of).

rhin- . . . **rhino-** . . . Greek combining forms, from *rhis,* genit. *rhinos* (nose), meaning *nose.*

rhino-kyph-osis. The condition of having a humped nose. / rhis, rhinos / kyphos (G. a hump) / osis (a noun-forming suffix denoting an *abnormal condition*).

rhiz- . . .   **rhizo-** . . .   Greek combining forms, from *rhiza* (a root), referring to a *root, spinal nerve root.*

rhizo-morph-ous. Resembling a root. / rhiza / morphe (G. form) / ous (an adjective-forming suffix meaning *marked by*).

rhod- . . .   **rhodo-** . . .   Greek combining forms, from *rhodon* (rose), meaning *rose, rose-red, red.*

rhod-ops-in. A pigment contained in the rods of the retina. / rhodon / ops (G. eye) / in (a noun-forming suffix used in *names of chemical compounds*).

rhythm- . . .   **rhythmo-** . . .   Greek combining forms, from *rhythmos* (rhythm), meaning *rhythm.*

a-rrhythm-ia. Lack of normal rhythm. / a (without) / rhythmos / ia (a noun-forming suffix used in names of *disorders*). *Note:* for duplication of the *r* in *arrhythmia,* see under *chyle-, chylor-rhea.*

ricketts- . . .   **rickettsi-** . . .   **rickettsio-** . . .   Combining forms, after Howard T. *Ricketts,* U.S. pathologist, referring to *rickettsia.*

rickettsio-gen-ous. Caused by rickettsiae. / Ricketts / gen (something that produces) / ous (an adjective-forming suffix meaning *having the power to*).

roentgen- . . .   **roentgeno-** . . .   Combining forms, after Wilhelm K. *Roentgen,* referring to *roentgen rays, x-rays.*

roentgeno-gram. An x-ray picture. / Roentgen / gramma (G. something written or depicted).

rostr- . . .   **rostri-** . . .   Combining forms, derived from the Latin *rostrum* (beak), referring to a *beak-like structure* or to a *beak.*

rostr-ate. Provided with a rostrum or beak. / rostr (beak) / ate (an adjective-forming suffix meaning *characterized by the presence of*).

rostri-form. Shaped like a beak. / rostri / form (a suffix meaning *in the shape of*).

-rrhage ... **-rrhagia** ... Greek combining forms, from *rhegnynai* (to burst), meaning *excessive flow, copious discharge*.

blenno-rrhagia. An excessive discharge of mucus. / blennos (G. mucus) / rrhagia. *Note:* for duplication of *r*, see under *chylorrhea*.

-rrhaphy ... A Greek terminal combining form, from *rhaphe* (a seam), referring to a *suturing, sewing together*.

teno-rrhaphy. The surgical suturing of a cut or torn tendon. / tenon (G. tendon) / rhaphe. *Note:* for doubling of *r*, see under *chylorrhea*.

-rrhea ... A Greek combining form, from *rhein* (to flow), referring to a *flow, discharge*.

leuko-rrhea. A whitish discharge from the vagina. / leukos (G. white) / rhein. *Note:* for duplication of the *r*, see under *chylorrhea*.

-rrhexis ... A combining form, derived from the Greek *rhexis* (a bursting), denoting a reference to a *rupture, bursting, break*.

onycho-rrhexis. The breaking of a nail. / onyx, genit. onychos (G. a nail) / rhexis (a breaking). *Note:* the *r* in *onychorrhexis* is doubled, in accordance with the rule that when a Greek word beginning with an aspirated *r* is preceded by a combining form ending in a short vowel, the *r* is doubled.

rube- ... **rubi-** ... **rubid-** ... **rubri-** ... **rubro-** ... Latin combining forms, from *ruber* (red) and *rubricatus* (reddened), meaning *red*.

rube-facient. A substance which reddens the skin. / ruber / facere (L. to make), present participle *faciens* (making), genit. *facientis*.

S

sacc- ... **sacci-** ... Latin combining forms, from *saccus* (a sac), meaning *sac, pouch.*

sacc-ate. Shaped like a sac. / saccus / ate (an adjective-forming suffix meaning *shaped like*).

-sacchar- ... **sacchari-** ... **saccharo-** ... Greek combining forms, from *sakcharon* (sugar), referring to *sugar, saccharum.*

saccharo-lysis. Decomposition of sugar. / sakcharon / lysis (L. a breaking up).

saccul- ... A Latin combining form, from *sacculus* (a small sac), referring to a *small sac.*

saccul-ar. Like a small sac. / sacculus / ar (a suffix forming adjectives meaning *like, of the nature of*).

-sacr- ... **sacro-** ... Latin combining forms, from *sacrum* (sacred), referring to the *sacrum, sacral bone. Note* the sacrum was formerly used in sacrifices.

sacr-alg-ia. Pain in the sacrum. / sacrum / algos (G. pain) / ia (a noun-forming suffix used in names of *disorders*).

-salping- ... **salpingo-** ... Greek combining forms, from *salpinx* (a trumpet), genit. *salpingos,* referring to a *uterine tube, an auditory tube.*

172

salping-emphraxis. An obstruction of a uterine tube or an auditory tube. / salpingos / emphraxis (G. an obstruction).

sangui-...   sanguin-...   sanguino-...   Combining forms, derived from the Latin *sanguis,* blood (genit. sanguinis), referring to *blood.*

sangui-col-ous. Living in the blood. / sanguis (blood) / colere (L. to inhabit) / ous (an adjective-forming suffix).

sapo-...   sapon-...   saponi-...   Latin combining forms, from *sapo* (soap), genit. *saponis,* referring to *soap.*

sapon-aceous. Having the qualities of soap. / saponis / aceous (a suffix meaning *having the characteristics of*).

sapr-...   sapro-...   Combining forms, derived from the Greek *sapros* (rotten), referring to *decay, putrefaction.*

sapro-phyte. A microorganism living on decaying matter. / sapros (rotten) / phyton (G. plant).

sarc-...   sarco-...   Greek combining forms, from *sarx,* genit. *sarkos* (flesh), referring to *flesh.*

sarco-lemma. The sheath surrounding a striated muscle fiber. / sarx, sarkos / lemma (G. a covering).

-scapul-...   scapulo-...   Latin combining forms, from *scapula* (shoulder), referring to the *scapula, shoulder blade.*

sub-scapul-ar. Beneath the scapula. / sub (beneath) / scapula / ar (an adjective-forming suffix meaning *pertaining to*).

scat-...   scato-...   Greek combining forms, from *skor,* genit. *skatos* (excrement), referring to *dung, fecal matter, excrement.*

scat-a-crat-ia. Inability to control the discharge of feces. / skor, skatos (feces) / a (without) / kratein (G. govern) / ia (a Latin noun-forming suffix used in names of *disorders*).

schist- ...   **schisto-** ...   Combining forms, derived from the Greek *schistos* (split), referring to a *cleft, fissure, split.*

schisto-gloss-ia. A condition in which the tongue is split lengthwise. / schistos (split) / glossa (G. tongue) / ia (a Latin noun-forming suffix used in names of *diseases* and *disorders*).

-schiz- ...   **schizo-** ...   Combining forms, derived from the Greek *schizein* (to divide), indicating *cleavage, division.*

schizo-trich-ia. Abnormal splitting of hair. / schizein (divide, split) / *thrix*, genit. *trichos* (hair) / ia (a Latin noun-forming suffix used in names of *diseases, disorders*).

-scler- ...   **sclero-** ...   Greek combining forms, from *skleros* (hard), referring to the *sclera of the eye.*

sclero-corne-al. Pertaining to the sclera and the cornea. / skleros / cornea tela (L. horny web, i.e. cornea of eye) / al (an adjective-forming suffix meaning *pertaining to*).

-scler- ...   **sclero-** ...   Greek combining forms, from *skleros* (hard), meaning *hard, fibrous.*

scler-osis. An abnormal hardening of a tissue or structure. / skleros / osis (a Greek noun-forming suffix denoting an *abnormal condition*).

scolio- ...   **scolioso-** ...   **scoliot-** ...   Combining forms, derived from the Greek *skolios* (crooked), carrying the concept of *curved, crooked, twisted.*

scolio-kyphosis. A lateral curvature of the spine associated with humpback. / skolios (crooked) / kyphosis (G. humpback).

-scope- ...   **scopo-** ...   **-scopy** ...   Greek combining forms, from *skopein* (to view), referring to *viewing, examining, inspecting, observing.*

endo-scope. An instrument used to examine the interior of the body or of an organ. / endo (from the Greek *endon*, within) /

scope (a suffix used to denote an examining instrument, from *skopein*).

scoto-...   A combining form, derived from the Greek *skotos* (darkness), denoting a relationship to *darkness, dark spot.*

scoto-phobia. Abnormal fear of darkness. / skotos (darkness) / phobos (G. fear). *Note:* the suffix *ia* is used in names of *diseases, disorders, conditions.*

scrot-...   scroto-...   Latin combining forms, from *scrotum* (a sac), meaning *scrotum.*

scroto-plasty. A plastic operation for the repair of the scrotum. / scrotum / plasty (a Greek terminal combining form meaning *plastic surgery involving a specified structure,* from *plastikos* (plastic), *plassein* (to form).

scyphi-...   scypho-...   Combining forms, from the Latin *scyphus* (cup) and the Greek *skyphos* (cup), referring to *a cup or cup-shaped structure.*

scypho-zoan. One of a class of sea coelenterates. / skyphos / zoion (G. animal).

seb-...   sebi-...   sebo-...   Latin combining forms, from *sebum* (tallow), meaning *sebum, fatty secretion.*

sebo-rrhe-al. Characterized by a discharge of sebum. / sebum / rrhea (from rhein, Greek for "to flow") / al (an adjective-forming suffix meaning characterized by). See note under *chylorrhea.*

-secret-...   secreto-...   Latin combining forms, from *secernere* (to separate, secrete), past participle *secretus* (separated, secreted), meaning *secretion.*

secreto-motor. Serving to stimulate secretion. / secretus / mot (from L. movere, to move, motus, past participle of movere) / or (a suffix denoting something that does a specified *function*).

-sect- ... **-section** ... **sectori-** ... Latin combining forms, from *secare* (to cut), past participle *sectus* (cut), referring to *a cutting, section.*

hemi-sect-ion. The act of cutting into two lateral halves. / hemi (half) / sectus (cut) / ion (a noun-forming suffix denoting an *action*).

secundi- ... **secundo-** ... Latin combining forms, from *secundus* (second), meaning *second, second time.*

secundi-para. A woman who has had two childbirths or who is having a second childbirth. / secundus, secunda / parere (to bear, give birth).

sediment- ... **sedimenti-** ... **sedimento-** ... Latin combining forms, from *sedimentum* (a sediment), referring to *sediment, sedimentation, precipitate.*

sedimento-gen-ic. Promoting the formation of a sediment. / sedimentum / gen (a Greek noun-forming suffix denoting *something that does* / ic (an adjective-forming suffix meaning *having a specified effect*).

selen- ... **seleno-** ... Greek combining forms, from *selene* (the moon), meaning *moon.*

seleno-graphy. The study of the features of the moon. / selene / graphia, graphein (G. to write, depict).

semi- ... A Latin prefix, from *semis* (half), meaning *half, partly, not fully.*

semi-lun-ar. Resembling a half-moon. / semis / luna (L. moon) / ar (an adjective-forming suffix meaning *of the nature of*).

semin- ... **semini-** ... **semino-** ... Latin combining forms, from *semen* (a seed), genit. *seminis*, referring to *semen, male reproductive fluid.*

semini-fer-ous. Carrying or conveying semen. / seminis / ferre

(L. to bear, carry) / ous (an adjective-forming suffix meaning *performing a specified function*).

sens-...   **sensi-**...   **senso-**...   **sensori-**...   Latin combining forms, from *sensus* (sense), meaning *sensation, sensory, sense.*

sens-orium. The seat of sensation in the brain; the whole sensory system. / sensus / orium (a Latin suffix denoting a place where something is situated).

sept-...   **septa-**...   **septi-**...   Latin prefixes, from *septem* (seven), meaning *seven, seventh.*

septi-gravida. A woman in her seventh pregnancy. / septem / gravida (L. woman heavy with child, from *gravis*, heavy).

-sept-...   **septi-**...   **septic-**...   **septico-**...   Greek combining forms, from *septikos* (putrefactive), referring to *putrefaction, decomposition, infection.*

septic-em-ia. The presence of bacterial products in the blood. / septikos / haima (G. blood) / ia (a noun-forming suffix used in names of *disorders*).

sept-...   **septo-**...   Latin combining forms, from *septum* (a hedge), meaning *septum, wall, partition.*

septo-tom-y. A surgical incision into a septum. / septum / tome (G. a cutting) / y (a noun-forming suffix denoting an action).

sero-...   A Latin combining form, from *serum* (whey), meaning *serum.*

sero-log-y. The science dealing with the properties and uses of serums. / serum / logos (G. word, study) / y (a noun-forming suffix denoting an *action, pursuit*).

sesqui-...   A Latin prefix, from *sesqui* (more by a half), meaning *one and a half.*

sesqui-cent-enni-al. A 150th anniversary; period of 150 years. /

sesqui / centum (L. a hundred) / annus (L. year) / al (a noun-forming suffix).

seta- ...   **seti-** ...   Latin combining forms, from *seta* (a bristle), meaning *bristle, stiff hair.*

set-aceous. Covered with bristles. / seta / aceous (a suffix meaning *characterized by, having*).

sex- ...   **sexi-** ...   Latin combining forms, from *sex* (six), meaning *six.*

sex-digit-ate. Having six digits. / sex / digitus (L. finger or toe) / ate (an adjective-forming suffix meaning *having*).

sexti- ...   **sextu-** ...   Latin combining forms, from *sextus* (sixth), meaning *sixth.*

sexti-par-a. A woman who has borne six children in six pregnancies. / sextus / parere (L. to bring forth) / a (a femine suffix).

-sial- ...   **sialo-** ...   Greek combining forms, from *sialon* (saliva), meaning *saliva.*

sialo-rrhea. An excessive flow of saliva. / sialon / rhein (G. to flow). See note under *chylorrhea.*

sialaden- ...   **sialadeno-** ...   Greek combining forms, from *sialon* (spittle, saliva) and *aden* (gland), referring to a *salivary gland.*

sialaden-itis. Inflammation of a salivary gland. / sialon / aden / itis (a suffix denoting *inflammation*).

sider- ...   **sidere-** ...   **sidero-** ...   Latin combining forms, from *sidus* (a star), genit. *sideris,* meaning *star.*

sidere-al. Pertaining to the stars. / sideris / al (an adjective-forming suffix meaning *pertaining to*).

sider- ...   **sidero-** ...   Greek combining forms, from *sideros* (iron), meaning *iron.*

sidero-penia. A deficiency of iron. / sideros / penia (G. poverty).

sigmoid-...   sigmoido-...   Greek combining forms, from *sigmoeides* (shaped like the letter S), referring to the *sigmoid flexure of the colon.*

sigmoido-scope. An instrument, a form of endoscope, used for examining the sigmoid. / sigmoeides / scope (an instrument for inspecting, from *skopein*, G. to see).

silic-...   silici-...   silico-...   Latin combining forms, from *silex* (flint), genit. *silicis*, meaning *silica, silicon.*

silic-osis. A form of lung disease caused by the inhalation of stone dust. / silicis / osis (a noun-forming suffix denoting an *abnormal condition*).

sinistr-...   sinistro-...   Latin combining forms, from *sinister* (left), meaning *left, left side.*

sinistr-ad. Toward the left. / sinister / ad (an adverbial suffix meaning *toward*).

sinus-...   sinuso-...   Latin combining forms, from *sinus* (a fold), meaning *sinus.*

sinuso-tom-y. A surgical incision into a sinus. / sinus / tome (G. a cutting) / y (a noun-forming suffix denoting an *action*).

-sis...   A noun-forming suffix, from the Greek *-esis*, denoting *a condition, activity.*

peristal-sis. The contractile movement of the intestine which propels the contents toward the point of expulsion. / peri (G. around) / stellein (G. to place) / sis.

sito-...   A Greek combining form, from *sitos* (food), referring to *food, eating.*

sito-phob-ia. Fear of food or eating. / sitos / phobos (G. fear) / ia (a Latin noun-forming suffix used in names of *disorders*).

sol-... solar-... solo-... Latin combining forms, from *sol* (the sun) and *solaris* (pertaining to the sun), referring to *sunlight, sun.*

sol-arium. A room suitable for exposing the body to the sun. / sol / arium (a variant of *-orium,* denoting a place).

som-... somat-... somatico-... somato-... Combining forms, derived from the Greek *soma,* genit. *somatos* (body), having reference to the *body* or *body build.*

som-a-sthen-ia. Weakness of the body. / soma (body) / a (without) / sthenos (G. strength) / ia (a noun-forming suffix).

somn-... somni-... somno-... Latin combining forms, from *somnus* (sleep), referring to *sleep.*

somn-ambul-ism. Sleep walking. / somnus / ambulare (L. to walk) / ism (a noun-forming suffix denoting an *act*).

-sophy... Greek terminal combining form, from *sophia* (wisdom), referring to *knowledge, wisdom, thought.*

theo-sophy. A religious system proposing the establishment of direct contact with divine principle through contemplation. / theos (G. god) / sophia.

sopor-... sopori-... Latin combining forms, from *sopor* (deep sleep), referring to *sleep, deep sleep.*

sopori-fic. Inducing sleep. / sopor / fic (an adjective-forming suffix derived from *facere,* to make).

span-... spano-... Greek combining forms, from *spanos* (scarce), meaning *scarcity, fewness.*

spano-meno-rrhea. Infrequent or scanty menstruation. / spanos / men (G. month) / rrhea (a suffix indicating a *flow*).

-spasm-... spasmato-... spasmo-... Greek combining forms, from *spasma* (a spasm), genit. *spasmatos,* meaning *spasm.*

pyloro-spasm. Spasm of the pylorus of the stomach. / pyloros (G. gatekeeper) / spasma.

speleo-... A Latin combining form, from *spelaeum* (a cave), referring to a *cave*.

speleo-logy. The scientific study of caves. / spelaeum / logia (G. study), from *logos*, word, study.

-sperm-... spermat-... spermato-... spermi-... spermo-... Greek combining forms, from *sperma* (seed), genit. *spermatos*, referring to *spermatozoa, sperm, seed*.

spermato-cyte. An early cell from which a spermatozoon develops. / spermatos / kytos (G. cell).

-sphen-... spheno-... Greek combining forms, from *sphen* (a wedge), meaning *wedge, wedge-shaped, sphenoid bone*.

spheno-cephal-y. A condition in which the head has a wedge-shaped appearance. / sphen / kephale (G. the head) / y (a noun-forming suffix denoting a *state, condition*).

spher-... sphero-... Greek combining forms, from *sphaira* (ball, sphere), meaning *sphere, spherical, round*.

sphero-cyte. A spherical red blood cell. / sphaira / kytos (G cell).

sphincter-... sphinctero-... Greek combining forms, from *sphinkter* (that which binds or draws close), referring to a *sphincter*.

sphinctero-plast-y. A plastic operation on a sphincter. / sphinkter / plastos (G. formed, from *plassein*, to form) / y (a noun-forming suffix denoting an *action*).

-sphygm-... sphygmo-... Greek combining forms, from *sphygmos* (pulse), meaning *pulse*.

sphygmo-mano-met-er. An instrument used for measuring blood

pressure. / sphygmos / manos (G. rare, thin) / metron (G. measure) / er (a noun-forming suffix denoting *a thing that performs a specified action*).

-spin- ...   **spini-** ...   **spino-** ...   Latin combining forms, from *spina* (backbone), referring to the *spine, spinal column, spinal cord.*

spini-fug-al. Conveying nervous impulses away from the spinal cord. / spina (spinal cord) / fugere (L. to flee) / al (an adjective-forming suffix imputing specified *characteristics*).

-spir- ...   **-spirat-** ...   **spiro-** ...   **-pir** ...   Combining forms, derived from the Latin *spirare* (to breathe), meaning *breathe, breathing.*

in-spir-ation. The act of breathing in. / in (a Latin prefix meaning *in*) / spirare (to breathe) / ation (a Latin noun-forming suffix denoting an *action*).

re-spirat-or. An apparatus used to administer artificial respiration. / re (L. again) / spiratus (past participle of spirare) / or (a Latin noun-forming suffix denoting a *person or thing performing a particular function*).

spirill- ...   **spirilli-** ...   **spirillo-** ...   Latin combining forms, from *spirillum* (a small coil), referring to the microorganisms known as *spirilla.*

spirill-em-ia. The presence of spirilla in the blood. / spirillum / haima (G. blood)/ ia (a noun-forming suffix used in names of diseases, disorders).

spirochet- ...   **spirocheti-** ...   **spirocheto-** ...   Greek combining forms, from *speira* (a coil) and *chaite* (a hair) i.e. a hairspring (in allusion to the shape of the microorganism), referring to *spirochetes.*

spirocheti-cide. A substance which kills spirochetes. / speira / chaite / cide (killer, from the Latin *caedere*, to kill).

splanchn-...   splanchnic...   splanchnico...   splanchno-
... Greek combining forms, from *splanchnon* (entrail) and *splanchnikos* (pertaining to entrails), meaning *viscera, viscus, organ.*

splanchn-ec-top-ia. The presence of a viscus or organ in an abnormal place. / splanchnon / ek (outside) / topos (G. a place) / ia (a noun-forming suffix used to denote a *disorder*).

-splen...   -spleni...   -spleno...   Greek combining forms, from *splen* (the spleen), referring to the *spleen.*

spleno-megal-y. Abnormal enlargement of the spleen. / splen / megale (G. large) / y (a noun-forming suffix indicating a *condition*).

spondyl-...   spondylo-...   Greek combining forms, from *spondylos* (vertebra), referring to a *vertebra, spinal column.*

spondyl-arthr-itis. Arthritis involving the joints between the vertebrae. / spondylos / arthron (G. joint) / itis (a suffix used to denote inflammation).

spongi-...   spongio-...   Greek combining forms, from *spongia* (sponge), referring to a *sponge, spongelike tissue, the corpus spongiosum.*

spongi-itis. Inflammation of the corpus spongiosum of the penis. / spongia / itis (a suffix used to denote *inflammation*).

-spor-...   -spore...   spori-...   sporo-...   Greek combining forms, from *spora* (seed), meaning *spore, reproductive cell.*

spor-angium. A capsule containing spores. / spora / angeion (G. a capsule).

-squam-...   squamat-...   squamo-...   Latin combining forms, from *squama* (scale), *squamatus* (provided with scales), referring to a *scale, squama, platelike structure.*

de-squam-ation. The shedding of scales; the shedding of the

skin in scales. / de (from, an undoing) / squama / ation (a noun-forming suffix denoting a *process*).

staped- . . .   **stapedi-** . . .   **stapedio-** . . .   Latin combining forms, from *stapes* (a stirrup), genit. *stapedis,* referring to the *stapes* of the middle ear.

staped-ec-tom-y. The surgical excision of the stapes. / stapedis / ek (out) / tome (G. a cutting) / y (a noun-forming suffix denoting an *action*).

staphyl- . . .   **staphylo-** . . .   Greek combining forms, from *staphyle* (a bunch of grapes), referring to the *uvula.*

staphyl-edema. A swelling of the uvula. / staphyle / oidema (G. a swelling, tumor).

staphylo- . . .   **staphylococc-** . . .   Greek combining forms, from *staphyle* (bunch of grapes) and *kokkos* (berry), referring to *staphylococci, staphylococcus.*

staphylo-cocc-em-ia. The presence of staphylococi in the blood. / staphyle / kokkos / haima (G. blood) / ia (a noun-forming suffix used in names of *diseases*).

stasi- . . .   **-stasis** . . .   **-static** . . .   Greek combining forms, from *stasis* (a standing), referring to *standing, arresting, being inactive.*

bacterio-stasis. Arrest of the growth of bacteria. / bakterion (G. a small staff) / stasis (arrest).

stear- . . .   **stearo-** . . .   **steat-** . . .   **steato-** . . .   Greek combining forms, from *stear,* genit. *steatos* (fat), meaning *fat, tallow.*

stearo-derm-ia. A disorder of the sebaceous or fat-producing glands of the skin. / stear / derma (G. skin).

stell- . . .   **stelli-** . . .   Latin combining forms, from *stella* (a star), meaning *star.*

stell-ate. Shaped like a star. / stella / ate (an adjective-forming suffix meaning *shaped like*).

steno-... A Greek combining form, from *stenos* (narrow), meaning *narrow, contracted, little.*

steno-pe-ic. Having a narrow opening or slit. / stenos / ope (G. opening) / ic (an adjective-forming suffix meaning *marked by*).

sterco-... stercor-... Latin combining forms, from *stercus*, genit. *stercoris* (dung), meaning *feces, stool, dung.*

stercor-oma. A mass composed of fecal matter. / stercus, stercoris / oma (G. swelling, tumor).

sterco-... A Greek combining form, from *stereos* (solid), meaning *solid, three-dimensional.*

stereo-gnosis. The ability to perceive the three-dimensional aspect and form of an object by touch. / stereos / gnosis (G. knowledge).

-stern-... sterno-... Greek combining forms, from *sternon* (sternum, breastbone), referring to the *sternum, breastbone.*

retro-stern-al. Behind the sternum / retro (behind) / sternon / al (an adjective-forming suffix meaning *pertaining to*).

steth-... stetho-... Combining forms, derived from the Greek *stethos* (chest), referring to the chest.

stetho-graph. An instrument used to record the movements of the chest. / stethos (chest) / graphein (G. record, delineate).

-sthen-... stheno-... Greek combining forms, from *sthenos* (strength), meaning *strength, vigor.*

hypo-sthen-ia. Decreased body strength. / hypo (decrease, below) / sthenos / ia (a noun-forming suffix used in names of *diseases, disorders*).

-stom- . . .   **stomat-** . . .   **stomato-** . . .   **-stomy** . .   Greek combining forms, from *stoma,* genit. *stomatos* (mouth), meaning *mouth, opening, pore.*

ozo-stom-ia. The condition of having a bad odor from the mouth. / ozo (G. an odor) / stoma / ia (a noun-forming suffix used in names of *disorders*).

strept- . . .   **strepto-** . . .   Greek combining forms, from *streptos* (twisted), meaning *twisted, twisted chain, curved*

strepto-coccus. A genus of microorganisms. / streptos (curved) / kokkos (G. berry).

strepto- . . .   **streptococc-** . . .   **streptococci-** . . .   **streptococco-** . . .   Greek combining forms, from *streptos* (twined, twisted) and *kokkos* (berry), referring to *streptococci, streptococcus.*

strepto-cocco-lys-in. A hemolysin produced by certain streptococci. / streptos / kokkos / lysis (G. a loosening) / in (a suffix used to designate certain *products*).

strepto-dermat-itis. Inflammation of the skin as a result of infection with streptococci. / streptos / derma (G. skin), genit. *dermatos* / itis (a suffix used to denote *inflammation*).

strictur- . . .   **stricturo-** . . .   Latin combining forms, from *stringere* (draw tight), past participle *strictus,* referring to a *narrowing, stricture.*

stricturo-tome. An instrument or surgical knife designed for cutting strictures. / strictus / tome (a suffix denoting a cutting instrument, from the Greek *tome,* a cutting).

stylo- . . .   A Latin combining form, from *stylus* (pillar, stake), referring to the *styloid process.*

stylo-mastoid. Pertaining to the styloid process of the temporal bone and to the mastoid process. / stylus / mastos (G. breast) / oeides (G. having the form of).

sub-... A Latin prefix, from *sub* (under), meaning *under, beneath, below, almost, near.*

sub-limin-al. Below the threshold, as of consciousness. / sub (below) / *limen* (L. threshold), genit. *liminis* / al (an adjective-forming suffix denoting a specified *characteristic*).

-sudor-... **sudori-**... **sudoro-**... Latin combining forms, from *sudor* (sweat), referring to *sweat, sweating, perspiration.*

sudori-fic. Causing perspiration. / sudor / fic (an adjective-forming suffix meaning *causing, making*, from the Latin *facere*, to make).

super-... A prefix, derived from the Latin *super*, above, used to indicate *above, higher, over, excessive.*

super-natant. Floating above or on the surface, as of a liquid. / super / natare (L. to swim).

super-son-ic. Having a speed above that of sound. / super / sonus (L. sound) / ic (an adjective-forming suffix).

supra-... A prefix, derived from the Latin *supra* (above), meaning *above, over, higher.*

supra-mastoid. Situated above the mastoid process of the temporal bone. supra / mastos (G. breast) / eidos (G. form). *Note:* the mastoid process was so named in allusion to its fancied resemblance to a breast.

syl-... A variant form of the Greek prefix *syn* (which see), used before combining forms beginning with the letter *l.*

syl-log-ism. A form of reasoning involving two premises and a conclusion. / syl (together) / logizesthai (G. to reason) / ism (a suffix indicating a *principle* or *theory*).

sym-... A variant form of the Greek prefix *syn* (which see), used before combining forms beginning with the letter *m.*

sym-phy-sis. A growing together or junction of bony parts. / sym (together) / phyein (G. to grow) / sis (a noun-forming suffix denoting a *process*).

sympath-... sympatheo-... sympathet-... sympathetic-... sympathetico-... Greek combining forms, from *sympatheia* (sympathy) and *sympathetikos* (sympathetic), referring to the *sympathetic nervous system, sympathetic nerve*. Note: *sympatheia* is derived from *syn* (together) and *pathein* (to feel).

sympathetico-ton-ia. Dominance, or excessive activity, of the sympathetic nervous system. / sympathetikos / tonos (G. tension) / ia (a noun-forming suffix denoting a *disorder*).

syn-... A Greek prefix, from *syn* (together), meaning *with, together, accompanying, associated with*. Note: *syn* changes to *syl* before the letter *l;* to *sym* before *b, m,* or *p;* to *sys* before an *s*.

syn-dactyl-y. A growing together of adjacent fingers or toes. / syn / daktylos (G. finger, toe) / y (a noun-forming suffix denoting an *action*).

synov-... synovi-... synovio-... Combining forms, from the Greek *syn* (with) and the Latin *ovum* (an egg), referring to *synovial fluid, synovial membrane*. Note: the etymology provides a likely allusion to the resemblance between synovial fluid and the white of an uncooked egg.

synovio-blast. A fibrous cell of a synovial membrane. / syn / ovum / blastos (G. a sprout).

syphil-... syphilo-... Greek combining forms, from *siphlos* (crippled), referring to *syphilis*.

syphilo-graphy. A treatise on syphilis. / siphlos / -graphia (writing, from the Greek *graphein*, to write).

syring-... syringo-... Greek combining forms, from *syrinx* (a tube), genit. *syringos*, referring to a *tube, fistula*.

syringo-myel-ia. The formation of cavities in the spinal cord. / syringos / myelos (G. marrow, spinal cord) / ia (a noun-forming suffix used in names of *diseases*).

sys-... A variant form of the Greek prefix *syn* (which see), used before combining forms beginning with the letter *s*.

sys-tol-e. Contraction of the heart. / sys (together) / stellein (G. to draw) / e (a suffix denoting an action).

systol-... **-systole...** **systolo-...** Greek combining forms, from *systole* (contraction), referring to the cardiac *systole*.

tele-systol-ic. Pertaining to the last part of a systole. / tele (G. far off) / systole / ic (an adjective-forming suffix meaning *pertaining to*).

T

tacho- ... **tachy-** ... Greek combining forms or prefixes, from *tachys* (swift), meaning *rapid, fast, swift*.

tachy-card-ia. A rapid beating of the heart; a fast pulse. / tachys / kardia (G. heart) / ia (a noun-forming suffix used in names of *disorders*).

-tact- ... **tacto-** ... Latin combining forms, from *tangere* (to touch), past participle *tactus*, meaning *touch, sense of touch*.

a-tact-il-ia. Absence of the sense of touch. / a (without) / tactus / ile (a suffix meaning *having to do with*) / ia (a noun-forming suffix denoting a *disorder*).

-tal- ... **talo-** ... Latin combining forms, from *talus* (ankle), referring to the *talus, ankle bone*.

talo-calcane-al. Pertaining to the talus and the calcaneus. / talus / calcaneum (L. heel bone) / al (an adjective-forming suffix meaning *pertaining to*).

-tars- ... **tarso-** ... **-tarsus** ... Greek combining forms, from *tarsos* (flat of the foot, any flat surface), referring to the *tarsus of the ankle, tarsus of eyelid*.

tarso-tibi-al. Pertaining to the tarsus and the tibia. / tarsos / tibia (L. shinbone) / al (an adjective-forming suffix meaning *pertaining to*).

tarso-malac-ia. An abnormal softening of the tarsus of the eyelid. / tarsos / malakos (G. soft) / ia (a noun-forming suffix used in names of *disorders*).

taur- . . .   **tauro-** . . .   Latin combining forms, from *taurus* (bull), referring to a *bull, ox.*

tauro-chol-ic. Pertaining to ox bile. / taurus / chole (G. bile) / ic (an adjective-forming suffix meaning *pertaining to*).

tauto- . . .   A Greek prefix, from *to auto* (the same), meaning *same, the same.*

tauto-phon-y. Repetition of the same sound. / to auto / phone (G. a sound) / y (a noun-forming suffix denoting an *action*).

-taxis . . .   **taxo-** . . .   Combining forms of Greek origin (*taxis*, agreement), referring to *order, orientation, arrangement.*

photo-taxis. Orientation of an organism, especially a plant, in response to the stimuli produced by light. / *phos*, genit. *photos* (G. light) / taxis (orientation, arrangement).

taxo-nom-y. The classification or arrangement of organisms. / taxo (order) / nomos (G. law) / y (a noun-forming suffix).

techn- . . .   **techno-** . . .   Greek combining forms, from *techne* (art), denoting *an art, craft, skill.*

techn-ician. A person skilled in the use of certain instruments or in the performance of tasks requiring training. / techne (art, skill) / ician (a suffix denoting a person specializing in a particular field).

tel- . . .   **tele-** . . .   Greek combining forms, from *tele* (far off), meaning *distant, far away.*

tele-ceptor. A nerve receptor which receives stimuli originating at a distance. / tele / ceptus (past participle of Latin capio, to take).

tel-... **tele-**... **telo-**... Greek combining forms, from *telos* (end), referring to an *end, termination, terminal.*

tel-angi-ectasis. Dilatation of end blood vessels. / telos (end) / angeion (G. vessel) / ektasis (G. stretching, dilatation).

-tempor-... **temporo-**... Latin combining forms, from *tempus* (temple), plural *tempora,* referring to the *temporal bone, temple.*

temporo-mandibul-ar. Pertaining to the temporal bone and the mandible. / tempora / mandibulum (L. jaw) / ar (a Latin adjective-forming suffix meaning *pertaining to*).

-tendin-... **tendino-**... **tendo-**... Latin combining forms, from *tendo* (tendon), genit. *tendinis,* referring to a *tendon.*

tendino-plast-y. A plastic operation on a tendon. / tendinis / plastos (G. formed) / y (a noun-forming suffix referring to an *action*).

teni-... **tenia-**... **tenio-**... Greek combining forms, from *tainia* (tape, ribbon), referring to *tapeworms.*

ten-iasis. The condition of being infested by a tapeworm. / tainia / iasis (G. a terminal suffix meaning *morbid condition*).

teno-... **tenon-**... **tenonto-**... Greek combining forms, from *tenon* (tendon), genit. *tenontos,* referring to a *tendon.*

tenonto-graphy. A treatise on, or a description of, tendons. / tenontos / -graphia (G. writing).

-tens-... **tensio-**... Latin combining forms, from *tensio* (tension), genit. *tensionis,* meaning *tension.*

tensio-meter. An instrument for measuring tension. / tensio / metron (G. measure) / er (a noun-forming suffix denoting something that performs a specified *function*).

hyper-tens-ion. An abnormally high blood pressure. / hyper (a

Greek prefix denoting excess, more than normal) / tensio / ion (a noun-forming suffix denoting a specified *condition*).

terat-...   terato-...   Greek combining forms, from *teras*, genit. *teratos* (monster), meaning *fetal monster*.

terat-ism. The condition of being a fetal monster. / teratos / ism (a noun-forming suffix indicating a *condition*).

terra-...   terri-...   Latin combining forms, from *terra* (earth), meaning *earth*.

terri-colous. Living in the earth or on the ground. / terra / colere (L. to dwell) / ous (an adjective-forming suffix).

terti-...   A Latin prefix, from *tertius* (third), meaning *third*.

terti-gravida. A woman who has been pregnant three times; a woman pregnant for the third time. / tertius / gravis, gravida (heavy, pregnant).

test-...   testi-...   testo-...   Latin combining forms, from *testis* (male gonad), referring to the *testes* or a *testis*.

testi-cond. A person having undescended testes. / testis / condere (L. to hide).

testicul-...   A Latin combining form, from *testiculus* (male gonad), referring to the *testicles* or a *testicle*. *Note: testiculus* is the diminutive of *testis*.

testicul-oma. A tumor of a testicle. / testiculus / oma (G. a tumor).

tetan-...   tetani-...   tetano-...   Greek combining forms, from *tetanos* (spasm), referring to *tetanus*.

tetani-gen-ic. Producing tetanus. / tetanos / gen (a combining form meaning "something that produces," from the Greek *gignesthai*, become) / ic (an adjective-forming suffix denoting a *specified characteristic*).

tetr- ...   **tetra-** ...   Greek combining forms, from *tettares* (four), meaning *four*.

tetra-dactyl-y. The condition of having four fingers or toes. / tettares / daktylos (G. finger) / y (a noun-forming suffix denoting a *condition*).

thalam- ...   **thalamo-** ...   Greek combining forms, from *thalamo*s (inner chamber), meaning *thalamus*.

thalamo-tom-y. The surgical destruction of a portion of the thalamus. / thalamos / tome (G. a cutting) / y (a noun-forming suffix denoting an *action*).

thalass- ...   **thalasso-** ...   Greek combining forms, from *thalassa* (the sea), meaning *sea*.

thalass-em-ia. A form of anemia occurring in peoples living along the Mediterranean Sea. / thalassa / haima (G. blood) / ia (a noun-forming suffix used to denote a *disorder*).

-thanas- ...   **thanat-** ...   **thanato-** ...   Combining forms, derived from the Greek *thanasimos* (murderous) and *thanatos* (death), denoting a reference to *death*.

eu-thanas-ia. An easy and painless death. / eu (G. well) / thanasimos (deadly) / ia (a Latin noun-forming suffix used to indicate a *condition*).

thanato-phob-ia. Abnormal fear of death. / thanatos (death) / phobos (G. fear) / ia.

thass- ...   **thasso-** ...   Greek combining forms, from *thassein* (to sit idle), meaning *idleness*.

thasso-phob-ia. Fear of being idle or unoccupied. / thassein / phobos (G. fear) / ia (a Latin noun-forming suffix used in names of *disorders*).

-thec- ...   **theco-** ...   Greek combining forms, from *theke* (sheath), meaning *case, sheath*.

theco-stegnosis. Narrowing of a tendon sheath. / theke / stegnosis (G. constriction, narrowing).

thel- . . .   **thele-** . . .   **thelo-** . . .   Greek combining forms, from *thele* (nipple), meaning *nipple.*

thel-itis. Inflammation of a nipple. / thele / itis (G. inflammation).

theo- . . .   A Greek combining form, from *theos* (god), meaning *diety, god.*

theo-phob-ia. Abnormal fear of God. / theos / phobos (G. fear) / ia (a Latin noun-forming suffix used in names of *disorders*).

therap- . . .   **therapeut-** . . .   **-therapy** . . .   Greek combining forms, from *therapeuein* (to treat) and *therapeutikos* (serving to heal), referring to *therapy, treatment.*

balneo-therap-y. The use of baths in the treatment of disease. / balneum (L. bath) therapeuein / y (a noun-forming suffix denoting an *action*).

-therm- . . .   **thermo-** . . .   **-thermy** . . .   Greek combining forms, from *therme* (heat), meaning *heat.*

hypo-therm-y. Low body temperature. / hypo (under) / therme / y (a noun-forming suffix denoting a *condition*).

-thigm- . . .   **thigmo-** . . .   Greek combining forms, from *thigma* (touch), referring to *touch, touch sensation.*

hypo-thigm-ia. A diminished sensitivity to touch. / hypo (a prefix indicating a decrease) / thigma / ia (a noun-forming suffix used in names of *disorders*).

thio- . . .   A Greek combining form, from *theion* (sulfur), referring to *sulfur.*

thio-phil-ic. Thriving in the presence of sulfur, as certain microorganisms. / theion / philein (G. to love) / ic (an adjective-forming suffix meaning *characterized by*).

thorac-...   thoracico-...   thoraco-...   Combining forms, derived from the Greek *thorax,* genit. *thorakos* (chest), referring to the *chest, thorax.*

thoraco-centesis. Surgical puncture of the chest wall. / thorax, thorakos (chest) / kentesis (G. puncture).

thromb-...   thrombo-...   Greek combining forms, from *thrombos* (a clot), meaning *thrombus.*

thrombo-lyt-ic. Tending to dissolve thrombi. / thrombos / lytikos (G. able to make loose) / ic (an adjective-forming suffix meaning *characterized by*).

thrombocyt-...   thrombocyto-...   Greek combining forms, from *thrombos* (clot) and *kytos* (cell), referring to *blood platelets.*

thrombo-cyto-penia. A decrease in the number of blood platelets. / thrombos / kytos / penia (G. poverty).

-thym-...   thymo-...   Greek combining forms, from *thymos* (the thymus), referring to the *thymus gland.*

thymo-privus. Designating a condition resulting from the removal of the thymus gland. / thymos / privus (L. deprived of).

-thymia...   thymo-...   Greek combining forms, from *thymos* (mind), meaning *mind, emotion, soul.*

thymo-genic. Caused by emotion. / thymos / genic (G. producing, from *gignesthai,* become).

thyro-...   thyroid-...   Greek combining forms, from *thyreoeides* (resembling a shield), referring to the *thyroid gland.*

hyper-thyroid-ism. Excessive activity of the thyroid gland and the disorder resulting from this. / hyper (excessive, abnormal) / thyreos (G. large shield) / eides (G. having form of) / ism (a suffix denoting a condition, usually abnormal).

tibi- ... **tibio-** ... Latin combining forms, from *tibia* (shinbone), referring to the *tibia*.

tibi-alg-ia. Pain in the shinbone. / tibia / algos (G. pain) / ia (a noun-forming suffix used in names of *disorders*).

-tion ... A noun-forming suffix, from the Latin *-tio, -tionis,* denoting *an act, process, condition, state.*

ab-lacta-tion. The weaning of a baby. / ab (off) / lactare (to suckle), past participle *lactatus* / tion.

-toc- ... **toco-** ... **toko-** ... Combining forms, derived from the Greek *tokos* (childbirth), referring to *childbirth, labor.*

dys-toc-ia. Difficult childbirth. / dys (a Greek prefix denoting *difficulty*) / tokos (childbirth) / ia (a Latin noun-forming suffix used in names of *disorders*).

-tom- ... **-tome** ... **tomo-** ... **-tomy** ... Combining forms, derived from the Greek *tomos* (piece cut off) or *temnein* (to cut), referring to a *cutting, surgical incision.*

micro-tome. An instrument for cutting thin sections of a tissue or other substance. / mikros (G. small) / temnein (to cut).

-ton- ... **tono-** ... Greek combining forms from *tonos* (tension), meaning *tone, tonus, tension.*

tono-met-er. An instrument for measuring tension. / tonos / metron (G. measure) / er (a suffix denoting a *thing that does*).

-tonsill- ... **tonsillo-** ... Latin combining forms, from *tonsilla* (tonsil), referring to *tonsils, tonsil.*

tonsill-ec-tom-y. The surgical excision of the tonsils. / tonsilla / ek (out) / tome (G. a cutting) / y (a noun-forming suffix denoting an *action*).

top-...   **topo-**...   Greek combining forms, from *topos* (place), meaning *place, region, area.*

top-a-gnosis. The inability to localize a touch sensation. / topos / a (without) / gnosis (G. knowledge).

torsi-...   **torsio-**...   **torso-**...   **torti-**...   Latin combining forms, from *torquere* (to twist), past participle *tortus* (twisted), referring to *rotation, twisting, turning.*

torti-coll-is. Wryneck. / tortus / collum (L. the neck) / is (a declensional suffix).

-tox-...   **toxi-**...   **toxico-**...   **toxo-**...   Greek combining forms, from *toxikon* (poison), referring to a *poison, toxin.*

tox-em-ia. The presence of poisonous substances in the blood. / toxikon / haima (G. blood) / ia (a noun-forming suffix denoting a *disorder*).

toxin-...   **toxini-**...   Combining forms, from the Greek *toxikon* (poison) and *in* (a suffix used in forming names for medicinal substances), referring to a *toxin, poison.*

toxini-cide. A substance which destroys a *toxin.* / toxikon / in / cide (a suffix meaning *killer*, from the Latin *caedere*, to kill).

-trache-...   **trachea-**...   **tracheo-**...   Greek combining forms, from *arteria tracheia* (rough artery, i.e. windpipe), referring to the *trachea, windpipe.*

tracheo-malac-ia. An abnormal softening of the trachea. / tracheia / malakos (G. soft) / ia (a noun-forming suffix used in names of *disorders*).

trachel-...   **trachelo-**...   Greek combining forms, from *trachelos* (neck), referring to the *neck, cervix.*

trachel-odyn-ia. Pain in the neck. / trachelos / odyne (G. pain) / ia (a noun-forming suffix used in names of *diseases*).

trans- ... A prefix, derived from the Latin *trans* (across), meaning *on the other side, through, beyond, across.*

trans-parent. Allowing the passage of light, and permitting a clear view of an object beyond. / trans (through) / parere (L. to appear), present participle *parens.*

trans-pleur-al. Performed through the pleura. / trans / pleura (G. side) / al (an adjective-forming suffix). *Note:* while the original meaning of the Greek word *pleura* is "side," it is used in this case to refer to the thin membrane covering the lung and lining the interior of the chest.

trauma- ... **traumat-** ... **traumato-** ... Greek combining forms, from *trauma,* genit. *traumatos,* (injury), meaning *injury, trauma.*

traumato-logy. The study of injuries. / traumatos / logia (G. study, from *legein,* to speak).

treponem- ... **treponemat-** ... **treponemi-** ... Greek combining forms, from *trepein* (to turn) and *nema,* genit. *nematos* (a thread), referring to *treponemes.*

treponem-iasis. Infection of the body with treponemes. / trepein / nematos / iasis (a suffix denoting a *morbid condition, infection, infestation*). *Note:* the semantic allusion of *trepein* and *nema* is directed toward the shape of the microorganism, which is that of a spiral or twisted thread.

tri- ... A Greek prefix, from *treis* (three), meaning *three, three times.*

tri-atom-ic. Composed of or containing three atoms. / treis / atomos (G. uncut, atom) / ic (an adjective-forming suffix meaning *characterized by*).

-trich- ... **tricho-** ... Greek combining forms, from *thrix,* genit. *trichos* (hair), meaning *hair.*

tricho-myc-osis. Infection of the hair with fungi. / trichos / mykes (G. fungus) / osis (a Greek noun-forming suffix indicating a *disorder*).

trichinell- ...   A Greek combining form, from *trichina* (a larval worm) and *ella* (a suffix denoting a diminutive form), referring to the worms of the genus *Trichinella*.

trichinell-iasis. Infestation with Trichinella organisms. / trichina / ella / iasis (a suffix denoting a *morbid condition, infestation*).

trichini- ...   **trichino-** ...   Greek combining forms, from *trichinos* (hairy), meaning *trichina*.

trichini-fer-ous. Bearing or containing trichinae. / trichinos / ferre (L. to bear) / ous (an adjective-forming suffix meaning *having, marked by*).

-tripsis ...   A Greek terminal combining form, from *tripsis* (a rubbing), referring to *rubbing, grinding, friction*.

odonto-tripsis. The wearing away of tooth substance by friction. / odous, odon (G. tooth), genit. odontos / tripsis (from *tribein*, to rub).

-trochanter- ...   **trochantero-** ...   Greek combining forms, from *trochanter* and ultimately from *trechein* (to run), meaning *trochanter*.

inter-trochanter-ic. Between the trochanters. / inter (L. between) / trochanter / ic (an adjective-forming suffix designating a *position*).

-trochle- ...   **trochleari-** ...   **trochleo-** ...   Latin combining forms, from *trochlea* (a pulley), meaning *trochlea, pulley*.

trochle-ar-i-form. Shaped like a trochlea or pulley. / trochlea / ar (an adjective-forming suffix meaning *like*) / i (a connecting particle) / forma (L. shape, form).

-trop- ... **-trope** ... **-tropia** ... **-tropic** ... **-tropism** ...
tropo- ... Greek combining forms, from *trope* (a turning),
denoting a *turning, changing, stimulating.*

trop-a-gnos-ia. The inability to perceive change in position. /
trope / a (not) / gnosis (G. knowledge) / ia (a noun-forming
suffix used in names of *disorders*).

-troph- ... **tropho-** ... **-trophy** ... Greek combining forms,
from *trophe* (food), referring to *nutrition, nourishment, food.*

myo-troph-ic. Providing nourishment to muscle tissue. / mys,
myos (G. muscle) / trophe / ic (an adjective-forming suffix).

trypan- ... **trpyano-** ... **trypanosom-** ... **trypanosomat-** ...
trypanosomato- ... **trypanosomi-** ... Greek combining
forms, from *trypan, trypaein* (to bore) and *soma* (body), referring to the microorganism *trypanosome.*

trypano-somi-cide. A substance destructive to trypanosomes. /
trypaein / soma / cide (a suffix meaning "killer," from *caedere,*
the Latin for "kill").

trypsin- ... **trypsino-** ... Greek combining forms, from
trypsis (a rubbing) and *in* (a suffix used to denote certain chemical compounds).

trypsin-ize. To treat with trypsin. / trypsis / in / ize (a verb-forming suffix meaning *cause to be*).

trypt- ... **trypto-** ... Greek combining forms, from *trypsis*
(a rubbing) and tic (an adjective-forming suffix used with
nouns ending in *sis*), referring to *trypsin.*

trypto-lyt-ic. Pertaining to the splitting action of trypsin. / lytos
(G. dissolved) / ic (an adjective-forming suffix meaning *characterized by*).

-tub- ... **tubo-** ... Latin combining forms, from *tubus* (a
pipe), referring to a *tube, uterine tube, auditory tube.*

tubo-abdomin-al. Pertaining to the uterine tubes and the abdomen. / tubus / abdomen (L. belly), genit. *abdominis* / al (an adjective-forming suffix meaning *pertaining to*).

tubercul- . . .   A Latin combining form, from *tuberculum* (nodule, small knob), referring to a *tubercle, tuberculosis*.

tubercul-ated. Covered with tubercles. / tuberculum / ated (a suffix denoting *possession of*).

tuberculo-derm. Tuberculous disease of the skin. / tuberculum / derma (G. skin).

tuberculin- . . .   **tuberculino-** . . .   Latin combining forms, from *tuberculum* (nodule, small knob) and -in (a suffix used to denote medicinal substances), referring to *tuberculin*.

tuberculin-ization. The application of tuberculin, as in testing for tuberculosis. / tuberculum / in / ization (a noun-forming suffix denoting a *process*).

tympan- . . .   **tympano-** . . .   Greek combining forms, from *tympanon* (drum), referring to the *eardrum, typmanum, middle ear*.

tympan-itis. Inflammation of the eardrum. / tympanon (eardrum) / itis (a suffix used to denote *inflammation*).

typhlo- . . .   A Greek combining form, from *typhlos* (blind), referring to *blindness*.

typhlo-phile. A person who is fond of and concerned about blind people. / typhlos / philein (G. to love).

typho- . . .   **typhoid-** . . .   Greek combining forms, from *typhos* (a vapor) and *eides* (resembling), referring to typhoid fever.

typho-bacter-in. A kind of typhoid vaccine prepared from dead bacteria. / typhos / bakterion (G. a small rod) / in (a suffix used to denote certain *medicinal preparations*).

U

ul-... uli-... ulo-... Greek combining forms, from *oule* (scar), meaning *scar, scar issue.*

ulo-gen-ous. Arising in scar tissue. / oule / gen (Greek suffix meaning *something that produces*) / ous (an adjective-forming suffix meaning *given to*).

ulcer-... ulcero-... Latin combining forms, from *ulcus* (ulcer), genit. *ulceris,* meaning *ulcer, sore.*

ulcero-gen-ic. Causing the formation of ulcers. / ulceris / gen (a suffix meaning *that which produces,* from the Greek *gignesthai,* become) / ic (an adjective-forming suffix meaning *characterized by*).

-ule... A noun-forming suffix, from the Latin *-ulus,* denoting *diminutive size, smallness.*

gran-ule. A small grain. / granum (L. a grain) / ule.

-ulent... An adjective-forming suffix, from the Latin *-ulentus,* meaning *full of, containing.*

corp-ulent. Having excessive fat or flesh. / corpus (L. body) / ulent.

ultra-... A prefix, derived from the Latin *ultra* (beyond), meaning *surpassing, beyond, excessively.*

ultra-micro-scop-ic. Too small to be seen by an ordinary microscope; beyond the range of an ordinary microscope. / ultra (beyond) / mikros (G. small) / skopein (G. to see) / ic (an adjective-forming suffix).

ultra-sonic. Beyond the range of perception by the human ear.
/ ultra / sonus (L. sound).

umbil- ...   **umbili-** ...   **umbilo-** ...   Latin combining forms,
from *umbilicus* (navel), meaning *navel, umbilicus.*

umbili-form. Resembling a navel. / umbilicus / forma (L.
shape, form).

un- ...   An Old English prefix meaning *not, negative, reversal.*

un-conscious. Insensible. / un / conscius (L. aware).

uni- ...   A Latin prefix, from *unus* (one), meaning *one.*

uni-foc-al. Having one focus. / unus / focus (L. hearth) / al
(an adjective-forming suffix).

-ur- ...   **-uria** ...   **urin-** ...   **urini-** ...   **uro-** ...   **urono-**
...   Greek combining forms, from *ouron* (urine), referring
to *urine.*

ur-em-ia. The presence of urinary impurities in the blood. /
ouron / haima (G. blood) / ia (a noun-forming suffix used in
names of *disorders*).

-ur- ...   **uro-** ...   Greek combining forms, from *oura* (tail),
referring to a *tail or tail-like structure.*

uro-pyg-ium. The hump at the rear end of a bird's body. / oura
/ pyge (G. rump) / ium (a suffix used to denote certain anatomical *structures*).

uranisco- ...   **urano-** ...   Greek combining forms, from
ouranos (vault of the sky), referring to the *palate, roof of the
mouth.*

urano-schism. The condition of having a cleft palate. / ouranos / schisma (G. a split).

-ure ... A noun-forming suffix, from the Latin *-ura*, denoting *result of an action, agency, instrumentality.*

junct-ure. A line or point of junction, as of two tissues. / jungere (L. to join), past participle *junctus* / ure.

urea- ... **ureo-** ... Greek combining forms, from *ouron* (urine), referring to *urea.*

ureo-tel-ic. Having urea as the end product. / ouron / telos (G. end) / ic (an adjective-forming suffix denoting a *characteristic*).

ureter- ... **uretero-** ... Greek combining forms, from oureter (urine canal), meaning *ureter.*

uretero-lysis. The freeing of a ureter from adhesions. / oureter / lysis (G. a loosening).

urethr- ... **urethro-** ... Greek combining forms, from ourethra (urethra), meaning *urethra.*

urethr-emphraxis. An obstruction of the urethra. ourethra / emphraxis (G. an obstruction).

uric- ... **urico-** ... Greek combining forms, from ourikos (pertaining to urine), referring to *uric acid.*

uric-acid-em-ia. The presence of an excessive amount of uric acid in the blood. ourikos / acidus (L. acid) / haima (G. blood) / ia (a noun-forming suffix used in names of *disorders*).

-uter- ... **utero-** ... Latin combining forms, from *uterus* (uterus), referring to the *uterus.*

utero-vesic-al. Pertaining to the uterus and the bladder. / uterus / vesica (L. bladder) / al (an adjective-forming suffix meaning *pertaining to*).

uve- ...   **uveo-** ...   Latin combining forms from *uva* (grape), referring to the *uvea* (choroid, ciliary body, and iris).

uve-itis. Inflammation of the uvea. / uva / itis (a suffix denoting *inflammation*).

uvio- ...   **uviol-** ...   Latin combining forms, from *ultra* (beyond) and *viola* (a violet), referring to *ultraviolet rays.*

uviol-ize. To subject to the effect of ultraviolet rays. / ultra / viola / ize (a verb-forming suffix meaning *treat with*).

uvul- ...   **uvulo-** ...   Latin combining forms, from *uvula* (small grape), meaning *uvula.*

uvulo-ptosis. An abnormal sagging of the uvula. / uvula / ptosis (G. a falling).

V

vacci- ... **vaccin-** ... **vaccini-** ... **vaccino-** ... Latin combining forms, from *vaccinus* (pertaining to a cow), referring to *vaccine*.

vacci-gen-ous. Producing a vaccine. / vaccinus / gen (that which produces, from the Greek *gignesthai*, become) / ous (an adjective-forming suffix meaning *characterized by*).

-vagin- ... **vagini-** ... **vagino-** ... Latin combining forms, from *vagina* (a sheath), meaning *vagina*.

vagin-ismus. A spasmodic contraction of the vagina. / vagina / ismus (L. an abnormal condition).

vago- ... A Latin combining form, from *vagus* (wandering, roaming), referring to the *vagus nerve*.

vago-ton-ia. Excessive activity of the vagus nerves. / vagari (L. to roam, wander) / tonus (L. a stretching, tension) / ia (a noun-forming suffix denoting a *disorder*).

valv- ... **valvi-** ... **valvo-** ... Latin combining forms, from *valva* (leaf of a folding door), referring to a *valve*.

valvo-tom-y. The surgical cutting of a valve. / valva / tome (G. a cutting) / y (a noun-forming suffix denoting an *action*).

valvul- ... **valvulo-** ... Latin combining forms, from *valvula* (a small door), referring to a *valve*.

207

valvulo-plasty. A plastic operation on a valve. / valvula / plasty (a suffix denoting a plastic operation, from the Greek *plastos,* formed).

vapo- ... **vapor-** ... Latin combining forms, from *vapor* (steam), referring to *vapor.*

vapo-therapy. The use of vapors in the treatment of disease. / vapor / therapeia (G. treatment).

varic- ... **varici-** ... **varico-** ... Latin combining forms, from *varix* (enlarged vein), genit. *varicis,* meaning *varix, dilated vein.*

varico-tom-y. A cutting into a varix. / varicis / tome (G. a cutting) / y (a noun-forming suffix denoting an *action*).

varicell- ... **varicelli-** ... Combining forms, derived from the Latin *varicella* (chickenpox), showing a relationship to *chickenpox.*

varicell-ation. Inoculation with chickenpox virus. / varicella (chickenpox) / ation (a Latin noun-forming suffix denoting a *process* or *action.*

variol- ... **varioli-** ... **variolo-** ... Latin combining forms, from *variola* (smallpox), referring to *smallpox.*

varioli-form. Resembling smallpox. / variola / forma (L. shape, form).

vas- ... **vasi-** ... **vaso-** ... Latin combining forms, from *vas* (a vessel), referring to a *blood vessel, lymph vessel, ductus deferens.*

vaso-con-strict-ion. The constriction or contraction of blood vessels. / vas / com, con (together) / strictus (L. bound) / ion (a noun-forming suffix used to denote a *process*).

vascul- ... **vasculo-** ... Latin combining forms, from *vasculum* (a small vessel), referring to a *blood vessel, vessel.*

vascul-ar-ization. The development of blood vessels in a tissue. / vasculum / ar (an adjective-forming suffix meaning *of the nature of*) / ization (a noun-forming suffix denoting a *process*).

ven-... **veni-**... **veno-**... Latin combining forms, from *vena* (vein), referring to a *vein, veins.*

intra-ven-ous. Situated in or involving the inside of a vein. / intra (inside, within) / vena / ous (an adjective-forming suffix meaning *affecting, involving*).

ventr-... **ventri-**... **ventro-**... Combining forms, derived from the Latin *venter,* belly, denoting a relationship to the *abdomen.* The combining forms are based on the genitive form *ventris.*

ventr-al. Pertaining to the abdomen; denoting the anterior aspect of the body. / ventr / al (an adjective-forming suffix).

ventro-scop-y. The medical examination of the interior of the abdomen with the aid of a special instrument. / ventr / o (combining particle) / skopein (G. to inspect) / y (a suffix forming nouns).

ventricul-... **ventriculo-**... Latin combining forms, from *ventriculus* (small belly), referring to a *heart ventricle, brain ventricle.*

ventriculo-puncture. A surgical puncture of a cerebral ventricle. / ventriculus / punctura (L. puncture, prick).

vermi-... **vermicul-**... Latin combining forms, from *vermis* (a worm) and *vermiculus* (a small worm), referring to a *worm.*

vermi-cide. A substance which kills worms. / vermis / cide (a suffix denoting something that kills, from the Latin *caedere,* to kill).

vermicul-ar. Resembling a worm or the movement of a worm. / vermiculus (a small worm) / ar (an adjective-forming suffix meaning *like*).

-vers-...   **versi-**...   **-version**...   Latin combining forms, from *vertere* (turn), past participle *versus,* meaning *turn, change.*

versi-color. Changing from one color to another. / versus / color (L. color).

-vertebr-...   **vertebro-**...   Latin combining forms, from *vertebra* (joint, vertebra), referring to a *vertebra.*

inter-vertebr-al. Situated between vertebrae. / inter (between) / vertebra / al (an adjective-forming suffix).

-vertigin-...   **vertigini-**...   **vertigino-**...   Latin combining forms, from *vertigo* (a turning around), genit. *vertiginis,* referring to *vertigo.*

anti-vertigin-al. Capable of checking vertigo. / anti (against) / vertiginis / al (an adjective-forming suffix meaning *characterized by*).

-vesic-...   **vesico-**...   Combining forms, derived from the Latin *vesica* (bladder), denoting a relationship to the *bladder.*

retro-vesic-al. Situated behind the bladder. / retro (L. behind) / vesica (bladder) / al (an adjective-forming suffix).

vesico-tom-y. A surgical incision into the bladder. / vesica / tome (G. a cutting) / y (a noun-forming suffix).

-vesic-...   **vesico-**...   Latin combining forms, from *vesica* (bladder), referring to a *blister, vesicle.*

vesic-ation. The formation of blisters. / vesica / ation (a noun-forming suffix denoting a *process*).

vesicul-...   **vesiculi-**...   **vesiculo-**...   Latin combining forms, from *vesicula* (a small bladder), referring to a *blister, vesicle.*

vesicul-itis. Inflammation of a seminal vesicle. / vesicula / itis (a suffix used to indicate *inflammation*).

vibrat- ...   **vibrato-** ...   **vibro-** ...   Latin combining forms, from *vibrare* (to vibrate), past participle *vibratus,* referring to *vibration.*

vibrat-ile. Capable of vibrating. / vibratus / ile (an adjective-forming suffix denoting *capability*).

vill- ...   **villi-** ...   **villus-** ...   Latin combining forms, from *villus* (tuft), referring to a *tuft, villus.*

vill-ose. Having villi. / villus / ose (an adjective-forming suffix meaning *provided with, having*).

vini- ...   A Latin combining form, from *vinum* (wine), meaning *wine, grapes.*

vini-fer-ous. Yielding wine. / vinum / ferre (L. to bear) / ous (an adjective-forming suffix meaning *characterized by*).

-vir- ...   **viri-** ...   **viril-** ...   **virili-** ...   Latin combining forms, from *vir* (man) and *virilis* (manly), meaning *male, man, masculine.*

viril-ism. Masculine characteristics in a female. / virilis / ism (a Latin noun-forming suffix denoting a *condition*).

-vir- ...   **viro-** ...   Latin combining forms, from *virus* (poison, slime), referring to *virus.*

viro-gen-ous. Caused by a virus. / virus / gen (a suffix meaning *produced by*) / ous (an adjective-forming suffix meaning *characterized by*).

virul- ...   **viruli-** ...   Latin combining forms, from *virulentus* (full of poison), referring to *virus, poison.*

viruli-cide. Something capable of killing a virus. / virulentus / cide (a suffix denoting something that kills, from the Latin *caedere,* to kill).

vis- ...   **visu-** ...   **visuo-** ...   Latin combining forms, from *videre* (to see), past participle *visus,* referring to *vision.*

visu-al-ize. To form a mental picture or image of something. / visus / al (an adjective-forming suffix meaning *having the characteristics of*) / ize (a verb-forming suffix meaning *to make*).

viscer- ... **visceri-** ... **viscero-** ... Latin combining forms, from *viscus* (organ), plural *viscera*, meaning *viscera, viscus, organ.*

viscero-ptosis. A sagging or drooping of organs. / viscera / ptosis (G. a falling).

-vit- ... **vita-** ... **vital-** ... Latin combining forms, from *vita* (life) and *vitalis* (marked by life), referring to *life.*

re-vital-ize. To restore to life; to return life to. / re (anew, again) / vitalis / ize (a verb-forming suffix).

-vitamin- ... **vitamino-** ... Latin combining forms, from *vita* (life) and *amine* (one of a group of compounds derived from ammonia), referring to *vitamins.*

hypo-vitamin-osis. An abnormal condition resulting from a deficiency of vitamins in the diet. / hypo (a prefix indicating a *decrease*) / vita / amine / osis (a noun-forming suffix used to denote a *disorder*).

-vitell- ... **vitelli-** ... **vitello-** ... Latin combining forms, from *vitellus* (yolk), referring to the *yolk of an egg or ovum.*

micro-vitell-ine. Having a small yolk. / mikros (G. small) / vitellus / ine (an adjective-forming suffix meaning *made of, having*).

vitr- ... **vitri-** ... Latin combining forms, from *vitrum* (glass), referring to *glass, glasslike substance.*

vitri-form. Having the appearance or form of glass. / vitrum / forma (L. form).

vivi- ... **vivo-** ... Combining forms, derived from the Latin *vividus* (lively), meaning *alive, living.*

vivi-section. The cutting of or experimentation on living animals. / vivi (alive) / secare (L. to cut).

vivo-sphere. The region, composed of the upper surface or layer of the earth and the lower portion of the atmosphere, where life exists. / vivo / sphaira (G. a ball or sphere).

-vorous... A Latin terminal combining form, from *vorare* (to eat), meaning *subsisting on, eating.*

carni-vor-ous. Eating mainly flesh. / caro (L. flesh), genit. *carnis* / vorare / ous (an adjective-forming suffix meaning *characterized by*).

vulv-... **vulvi-**... **vulvo-**... Latin combining forms, from *vulva* (a covering, womb), referring to the *vulva, female genitals.*

vulv-itis. Inflammation of the vulva. / vulva / itis (a suffix used to denote *inflammation*).

X Y Z

xanth-...   xantho-...   Greek combining forms, from *xanthos* (yellow), meaning *yellow*.

xantho-chrom-ia. An abnormal yellowing discoloration. / xanthos / chroma (G. color) / ia (a noun-forming suffix used to denote a *disorder*).

xeno-...   A Greek combining form, from *xenos* (foreign), meaning *foreign, foreign body, stranger*.

xeno-phob-ia. An abnormal dislike for strangers. / xenos / phobos (G. fear, dislike) / ia (a Latin noun-forming suffix used in names of *disorders*).

xero-...   A combining form, derived from the Greek *xeros* (dry), indicating *dryness*.

xero-cheil-ia. Abnormal dryness of the lips. / xeros (dry) / cheilos (G. lip) / ia (a Latin noun-forming suffix used in names of disorders).

xiph-...   xiphi-...   xipho-...   Greek combining forms, from *xiphos* (a sword), referring to the *xiphoid process of the sternum*.

xiph-oid-itis. Inflammation of the xiphoid process. / xiphos / eides (G. like) / itis (a suffix used to denote *inflammation*).

xyl-... xylo-... Greek combining forms, from *xylon* (wood), referring to *wood.*

xylo-carp-ous. Bearing woody fruit. / xylon / karpos (G. fruit) / ous (an adjective-forming suffix denoting a *characteristic*).

-y... A noun-forming suffix, from the Latin *ia,* denoting *a condition, quality, result of an action.*

obesit-y. The condition of being fat. / obedere (L. to devour), past participle *obesus* / y.

zo-... zoo-... Combining forms, derived from the Greek *zoion* (animal), referring to *animals* or *animal life.*

zo-anthrop-y. A mental disorder in which the patient believes that he is transformed into an animal. / zo (animal) / anthropos (G. man) / y (a noun-forming suffix denoting a condition).

zoo-phag-ous. Eating animal food. / zoo (animal) / phagein (G. to eat) / ous (an adjective-forming suffix).

zyg-... zygo-... Greek combining forms, from *zygon* (a yoke), meaning *pair, paired, joined, junction.*

a-zyg-ous. Not paired. / a (not) / zygon (yoke) / ous (an adjective-forming suffix denoting a *characteristic*).

zygo-dactyl-y. A fusion of fingers or toes. / zygon / daktylos (G. finger) / y (a noun-forming suffix meaning a *condition*).

zygomatic-... zygomatico-... Greek combining forms, from *zygomata* (the plural form of *zygoma,* a bar) and the adjective-forming suffix *-ic* (pertaining to), referring to the *zygoma, zygomatic arch, zygomatic bone, zygomatic process. Note: zygomatic* may also be regarded as derived from *zygoma* and *-tic* (an adjective-forming suffix meaning *pertaining to*).

zygomatico-maxill-ary. Pertaining to the zygoma and the maxillary bone. / zygomata / ic / o (connecting vowel) / maxilla (diminutive of the Latin *mala,* upper jawbone) / ary (an adjective-forming suffix meaning *pertaining to*).

-zymo- ...   A Greek combining form, from *zyme* (ferment), referring to *ferments, fermentation, enzymes.*

zymo-phyte. A microorganism causing fermentation.   zyme / phyton (G. plant).

zymo-phore. The active group of an enzyme molecule. / zyme / phore (G. bearer, from pherein, to bear).